ADVANCE PRAISE FOR

The Magic Ten and Beyond

"*The Magic Ten and Beyond* is a brilliant formula for anyone who wants to start their day in an auspicious and blessed way. Sharon's teaching style infuses the practice with pure magic and love. This collection of inspired yogic gems is a treasure chest filled with spiritual gold. I highly recommend checking out this awesome book!"

—MC YOGI, musician and author of *Spiritual Graffiti: Finding My True Path*

"As a physical therapist, yoga teacher, and anatomy instructor, I teach and encourage my clients and doctoral students to learn the Magic Ten Asana Sequence and to do it regularly. It is an easy, reproducible practice that increases overall strength and flexibility, while moving your spine in all the six directions required for optimal mobility. In addition, the Magic Ten provides range of motion for the joints that aren't always accessed in a typical workday. You will be stronger, more mobile, and healthier doing this practice daily. The U.S. Department of Health and Human Resources suggests that we all do 150 minutes of moderate exercise a week in at least ten-minute bouts. I have found that the Magic Ten fits nicely into a ten-minute bout of exercise. Having benefited from the Magic Ten for years, I am looking forward to incorporating the other practices that Sharon shares in her new book, *The Magic Ten and Beyond*."

—DR. LORI ZUCKER, PT, DPT, CYT

"As a classical musician, I spend 75 percent of my time traveling the world performing. If it wasn't for the Magic Ten and Beyond sequences, which I do every morning along with the vegan diet that Sharon recommends, I would not have the strength and focus I need as a performer. Since following her practical Magic Ten and Beyond, I have experienced reduced stress while traveling, suffer almost no jet lag, feel completely present in each new environment, and have a new sense of effortlessness when performing."

—KATYA GRINEVA, internationally acclaimed concert pianist
and winner of the Gusi Peace Prize

"The practices in *The Magic Ten and Beyond* have helped me create a life filled with joy, well-being, and connection. Sharon is one of my greatest teachers, and in this book she shares simple tools that will radically transform your life for the better. Plus, these practices are easy to do and don't take long at all! Use them on a regular basis and watch how you begin to effortlessly flow with the abundant energy of life."

—KRIS CARR, *New York Times* bestselling author, cancer thriver, and wellness activist

"*The Magic Ten and Beyond* is a wonderfully inspired instructional on how to use our bodies, breath, and personal intention as daily *sadhana*, or spiritual practice. It is also an embodied alchemical ritual designed to transform the 'lead' of our ego and attachments into the 'gold' of our ever-evolving consciousness. Magic is about shifting our energetic realities at will and through detailed instruction Sharon guides us to experience these changes within ourselves. Through weekly reflection, meditation, and asana practice, developed to support us in our personal investigation of Self, we can experience the powerful *magic* that is within our own being and witness the ways these transformations affects our life. I highly recommend this thoughtful book to anyone looking for meaning and inspiration in their practice that can take them beyond their body and into the very heart of their Spirit."

—SEANE CORN, yoga teacher and cofounder of Off the Mat, Into the World

"I am grateful for *The Magic Ten and Beyond*. It is a wonderful collection and practical template for one's personal *sadhana*. All of the practices revealed in this powerful book are extremely effective and have helped keep me on the path, informed my life, and strengthened me. Sharon is a guiding light, a wonderful teacher, and a great storyteller. I relate to her instincts on Ancient Egypt and its connection to Yoga as well as her practical advice on vegan living. Kudos to Guzman, as well—the photographs are beautiful."

—ROB FRABONI, Grammy Award–winning music producer, former vice president of Island Records, and inventor of RealFeel ™ audio technology

"Sharon Gannon has crafted for us a doable series of life-affirming and soul-satisfying disciplines drawn from both ancient teachings and the insights she gains daily doing these practices herself. And her gentle, add-as-you-go approach makes this transformational process accessible to busy people and even to spiritual skeptics."

—VICTORIA MORAN, author of *Main Street Vegan*, *The Good Karma Diet*, and *Creating a Charmed Life*

"If you're a seeker who resonated with *The Artist's Way*, this book will transform the way you think of your spiritual path. *The Magic Ten and Beyond* is a necessary guide to deepen our relationship to yoga, God, and ourselves. Sharon's easy-to-follow practices and options breathe life into how we can live fully and compassionately on and off the mat."

—KIMBERLY WILSON, therapist, author, and yogi at kimberlywilson.com

"*The Magic Ten and Beyond* is the yogi's way to go. All of the practices in this book are tangible and doable and have the power to transform us from violence to nonviolence. If you take any one of the chapters and fully incorporate the practice into your life, magic will happen. That magic ripples from your own being to the hearts and souls of all beings. Sharon is the perfect person to lead this movement. Where she leads, I will follow with eyes wide open."

—COLLEEN SAIDMAN-YEE, author of *Yoga for Life*

ALSO BY SHARON GANNON

Cats and Dogs Are People Too!

Jivamukti Yoga: Practices for Liberating Body and Soul (with David Life)

The Art of Yoga (with David Life)

Yoga and Vegetarianism: The Diet of Enlightenment
(translated into seven languages)

Yoga Assists (with David Life)

Simple Recipes for Joy: More than 200 Delicious Vegan Recipes

THE MAGIC TEN AND BEYOND

DAILY SPIRITUAL PRACTICE FOR
GREATER PEACE AND WELL-BEING

SHARON GANNON

A TarcherPerigee Book

tarcherperigee

An imprint of Penguin Random House LLC
375 Hudson Street
New York, New York 10014

Photo and illustration credits:

All photos of Sharon Gannon by Guzman except where noted

All illustrations by David Life, except where noted

Page 53: Life, David. Egyptian Yogini Sitting in Virasana Practicing Pranayama. Watercolor painting, 2016

Page 68: Gannon, Sharon. Admission ticket to the Great Pyramid, 2008

Page 69: Life, David. Sharon lying in the coffer of the Great Pyramid, 2008

Page 71: Life, David. Egyptian Yogini. Watercolor painting, 2017, after an Egyptian painting on stone from 1200 BCE

Page 79: House Shrine, Pharaoh Akhenaten, his queen Nefertiti, and their three daughters being blessed by the Aten. Amarna period, ca. 1340 BCE, carved limestone relief. Egyptian Museum, Berlin. Photograph of relief taken by the author, 2016

Page 84: Life, David. Cartouche. Watercolor painting, 2016

LIBRARY OF CONGRESS CATALOGING-IN-PUBLICATION DATA
Names: Gannon, Sharon, author.
Title: The magic ten and beyond : daily spiritual practice for greater
peace and well-being / Sharon Gannon.
Description: First edition. | New York : TarcherPerigee, 2018. | "A
TarcherPerigee book."
Identifiers: LCCN 2017053400 (print) | LCCN 2018003469 (ebook) | ISBN
9780143131441 (E-book) | ISBN 9781524705176 (pbk.)
Subjects: LCSH: Yoga. | Spiritual life.
Classification: LCC BL1238.52 (ebook) | LCC BL1238.52 .G36 2018 (print) | DDC
204/.4—dc23
LC record available at https://lccn.loc.gov/2017053400

Printed in the United States of America

3 5 7 9 10 8 6 4

Book design by Pauline Neuwirth

CONTENTS

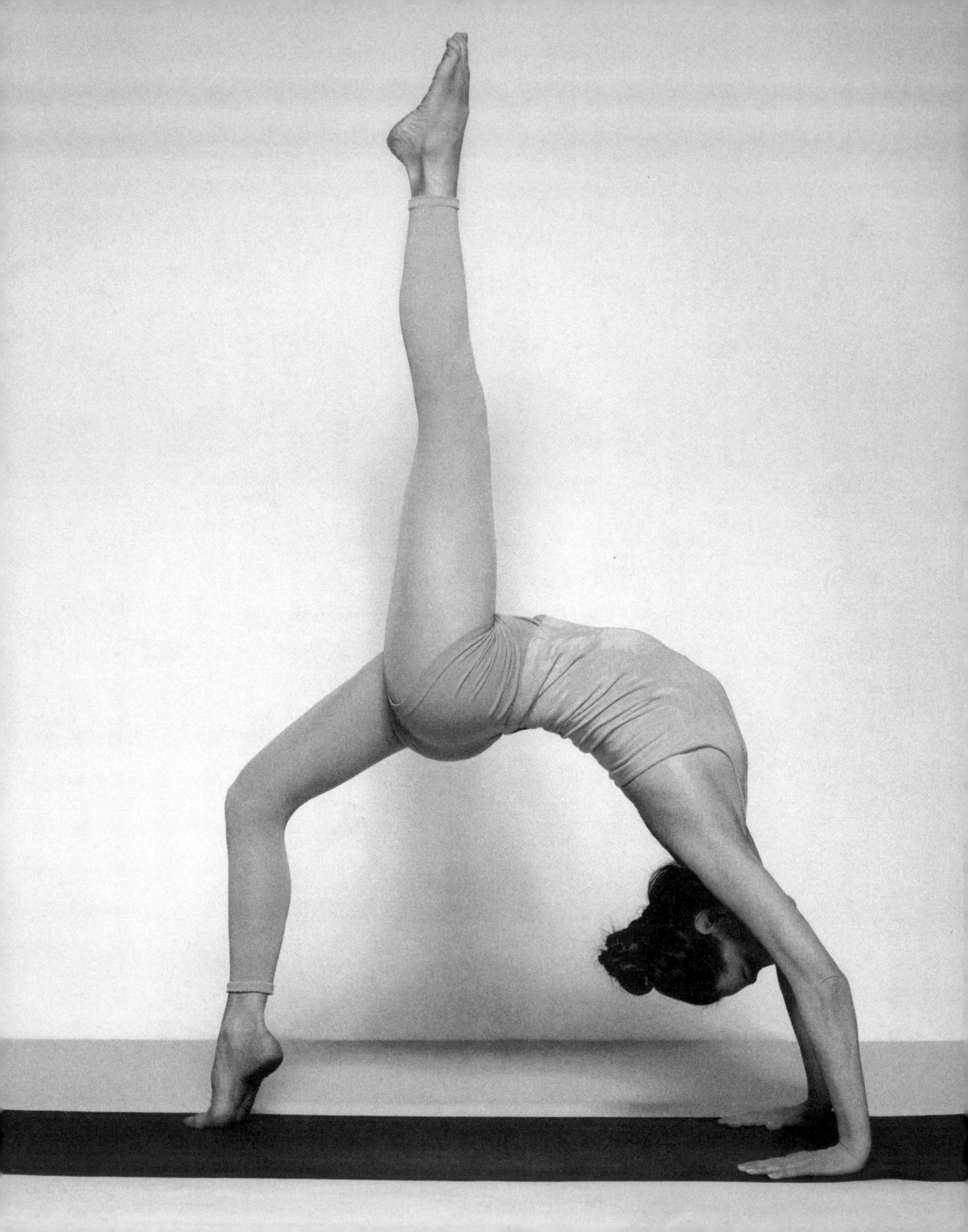

INTRODUCTION TO THE WAY

YOGA IS A SANSKRIT WORD that means "to yoke or reconnect," and it refers to both the practice and the goal of the practice. The goal of yoga is Yoga—to remember one's connection to the Supreme Source, eternal happiness itself. Yoga teaches that within each living being there is an eternal soul, the atman. The practices enable us to reconnect to the atman and to understand that our mortal bodies are dwelling places for our immortal soul. The practices alchemically transform our perception of who we are. The body of the enlightened yogi houses the light of truth. The yogi lives in the world as an instrument for this truth. There are many yoga practices that can guide a person along the way to that magical remembering of who he or she really is. Some of those practices are explored in this book.

There are accounts in the various yogic scriptures and holy books from India that describe the path, or way, of yoga. We can read about the lives of great yogis from ancient times and get a glimpse into their world and into how they walked their paths. In this book I share some of the practices that have helped me along my way. I also share some of my ideas regarding the history of yoga and my speculations regarding its possible connection with ancient Egypt. I love India and have great respect for the spiritual wisdom of her culture, and yet I can't deny that I am attracted to the mysteries of ancient Egypt and feel that yoga may be more universal than is usually thought and could have been shared by both cultures. Ten years ago this intuition led me to visit Egypt. While in the Great Pyramid, lying in the King's Chamber, I had an out-of-body experience. A day later at the Egyptian Museum in Cairo I saw a painting of a figure that looked as if she were doing an asana (see page

71), and met an Egyptologist who showed me a magic circle, called a cartouche (see page 84), containing ten hieroglyphs that looked to me like they could be describing yoga practices—remarkably, the ten practices I did every morning.

This is why every chapter begins with an image of an Egyptian hieroglyph followed by a poetic account as to how the meaning of the hieroglyph might translate into the yoga practice described. The practices that make up the ten-week course will certainly stand alone, but if you want to delve deeper and learn more about the hieroglyphs as well as the backstory, "A Story," found on page 67, tells of my yoga adventure in Egypt and its connection to the *sadhana* shared in this book.

The Sanskrit word *sadhana* means "conscious spiritual practice." What distinguishes a yoga practice from a physical fitness exercise routine is intention. When you engage in an activity with the conscious intention for it to bring you closer to enlightenment—to the realization of the oneness of being—then it is sadhana. Sadhana is never something you do for yourself. It is always about getting *over* yourself, your separate ego self, and awakening to how you are part of a higher Divine Self. Without the essential ingredient of *bhakti*, which means "devotion or love for God," sadhana will not yield anything interesting or magical but instead will keep one ego-centered and bound in mundane reality and the pursuit of temporary happiness through material accumulation.

With yoga centers in just about every city, town, and village in the world today, a person has many opportunities to take yoga classes and to study with qualified teachers. I am not advocating for rejecting the yoga studio model, but we should nonetheless remember that yoga is about reconnecting to God, which is ultimately a solitary journey inward. As yogis we should develop independence—dependence inward. The journey within is the journey toward lasting happiness. To be able to go to a class with others is great, and it has many benefits. But sometimes, whether because of schedule demands or financial limitations, attending a yoga class may not be possible. That shouldn't mean that you can't practice yoga. You should have something easy and doable that you can access any time, so that you are not dependent on going to a class to practice yoga, and yoga can become a way of everyday life. Traditionally, yogis learned under the tutelage of a teacher, but then continued their practice privately on their own.

I love going to yoga classes, but it is often not practical for me to do so. I practice on my own every day. My practice starts in the morning when I wake up, while I am still lying in bed, as I remember to be grateful. What I reveal in this book is how my practice continues to unfold from there, how my personal sadhana—which I have done over the years in the privacy of my home or in a hotel room or wherever I happen to be—provides me with a way that launches me into the day and hopefully helps me to be a better, kinder, calmer, more spiritual person.

The Magic Ten and Beyond is my way of sharing that sadhana. The ten practices are presented as a ten-week course, providing the beginner as well as the seasoned yogi with a how-to formula for a home practice. They can be done together as a standalone practice or as a warm-up—a preparation for a longer, more complete asana practice.

There are practices for how to wake up in a good mood every morning and for how to become more saintly; practices that reveal the secrets to wealth and abundance and that will increase your vital energy by teaching you how to conserve and direct your *prana*, or life force. There are practices that will help you resolve old relationship issues by detoxifying your body and purging your thoughts of negative emotions, and that will keep you limber and fit well into old age. There is an easy step-by-step meditation practice as well as a way to free yourself from the fear of death and live at ease comfortably in your own skin for the rest of your life.

THE WAY TO USE THIS BOOK

FOR A PRACTICE TO YIELD sweet fruit it must be done regularly—daily is best. It should become a habit, a good habit like brushing your teeth. And like brushing your teeth, a daily yoga practice doesn't have to take all day. Do it first thing in the morning and allow the benefits to unfold and reveal themselves throughout the rest of the day. Over time, with consistent regular daily practice, the benefits will accumulate. Transformation is always subtle and gradual, but nonetheless inevitable, if you commit to consistency in your practice.

The book is divided into chapters or weeks. Each chapter's heading shows "the way"—a focused introduction to a specific practice—followed by practical instructions for how to do the practice for that week. There is also a glossary at the end of the book, to help you understand many of the Sanskrit and other foreign terms that are used throughout the book.

> *Option #1:* Utilize the book to provide you with a practice that gradually increases in intensity from week to week over a ten-week period. For example, for the first week, every day you practice "Gratitude." In the second week, you add the practice of "Giving Blessings." Third week, you add "Feeding the Birds," and you keep going, adding a new practice each week. At the end of Week 10 you will be doing all the ten practices in sequence every day.

Option #2: Take any of the practices that appeal to you and practice them à la carte.

Option #3: Select just the "Magic Ten" series of asanas that appear in Week 4, Connecting the Way—a simple physical practice that can be done in about ten minutes that will keep your body fit and limber.

Option #4: Use all ten practices or any of them as a prelude or warm-up for your own asana practice. If you choose this option, it is best to place the practice of *shavasana*—deep relaxation, given in Week 10—after your asana practice.

Option #5: Customize and rearrange the sequence of the practice into a different order than is presented in the book. For example, sit down to meditate first thing in the morning, shifting practice 9 to the number 1 spot. Afterward, let the sequence unfold as you practice gratitude, giving blessings, feeding the birds, and so forth.

Always feel free to creatively modify the practices so that they fit your capacity and lifestyle. As you will see, I have provided some suggested options to help with that. Do your best and leave the rest, or, as I like to say, "Do your best and let God do the rest."

• WEEK 1 •

AWAKENING THE WAY

GRATITUDE

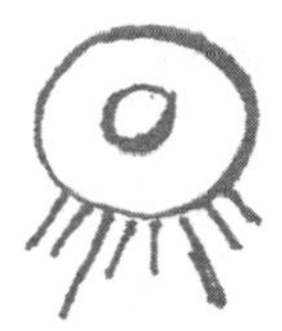

WEEK 1—Awakening the Way: Gratitude

The sun, in a kind and caring way, extends life-giving rays to all living beings on Earth, providing us with warmth, light, and life—the energy that lifts us upward to our fuller potential as kind and caring beings.

Life is a privilege. Humility is a most important virtue to cultivate for the yogi because through humility one can diminish self-centeredness and awaken to Self-realization. With each new day we are given an opportunity to remember who we really are—to remember our divine, eternal connection to the Supreme. Gratitude awakens humility, and humility leads to enlightenment. How you begin your day will color your whole day. If you want the presence of goodness to guide you throughout your day, the best way is to remember the source of goodness as soon as you wake up. To wake up in a good mood is something that you can actually train yourself to do. That is what a practice is; it is not something that necessarily comes naturally. At the beginning conscious training is essential. Over time your discipline will begin to yield results, the practice will become second nature, and you will gracefully wake up in the mood of gratitude.

Yoga means "to remember God." Most of us wake up in the morning with thoughts about ourselves and with questions like, "What am I going to do today?" Right away we get busy with planning what we are going to do, and with those thoughts we forget the actual source of our doing. When we forget God we focus on ourselves as the doer, and that can feel quite overwhelming when we face all the things we have to do—the problems we feel we have to fix at home, at work, and in the world. We may even fall into the habit of complaining about our lives, other people who are creating obstacles for us, and the unfairness of it all. Complaining actually rewires your brain—the more you complain, the easier it is to complain, and over time you find yourself in a negative spiral. The antidote for the poison of complaining is gratitude. If we can mindfully catch ourselves when we are about to fall into complaining and instead lift ourselves up by finding something to be grateful for, we will be able to break the negative habit of complaining, which leads to self-loathing, worry, anxiety, and fear about getting up in the morning. Through gratitude we experience humility: we offer ourselves as instruments for the will of the Supreme Self so that we may relax and participate as players in the creative unfolding of the great mystery that is life.

Many people might find it difficult to relate to God, but the force of God, or what one may call the enlightenment principle or the power of unconditional love, comes through in many tangible forms—as gurus or teachers. Anyone can be our teacher. Our parents are our first teachers. It is up to us to see the teacher in another person, decide to treat them with respect, and listen to the messages they give. In our journey through life, if we are open to hearing others, we will encounter teachers who will provide the right guidance and will help us remember who we really are. Feeling gratitude for their presence in our lives is a powerful way to cultivate humility and bring us closer to Yoga—to enlightenment.

THE PRACTICE

As soon as you wake up, while still lying in bed, aloud or silently say a prayer that expresses gratitude for your life, gratitude for being given an opportunity to remember God, and the desire to be kind to others.

Option #1: Thank God for this day. Say, "Everything I do today, every action, I offer to you, my Lord, may Your bliss increase in this world. Please accept my offering."

Option #2: Chant the Sanskrit pledge: *"Lokah Samasta Sukhinoh Bhavantu."* Or say it in English: "May all beings everywhere be happy and free and may the thoughts, words, and actions of my own life contribute in some way to that happiness and to that freedom for all."

Option #3: Ask your higher Self to make you His or Her instrument. Say, "Make me an instrument for Thy will—not mine but Thine be done. Free me from anger, jealousy, and fear; fill my heart with joy and compassion."

Option #4: Express gratitude for the teachers in your life. Remember the good things that they have done for you and for others. Talk to them, address them by name, and thank them for being in your life.

Option #5: Chant the traditional Sanskrit mantra to the guru, from the *Guru Strotam*: *"Guru Brahma, Guru Vishnu, Guru Devo Maheswara, Guru sakshat, param Brahma, tasmai shri guruvey namah, tasmai shri guruvey namah."* Or say it in English: "Our creation is that guru; the duration of our lives is that guru; our trials, illnesses, and calamities are that guru; there is a guru that is nearby and a guru that is beyond the beyond. I humbly make my offering to the guru, the beautiful remover of ignorance, the enlightenment principle that is within me and surrounds me at all times."

• WEEK 2 •

BLESSING THE WAY

GIVING BLESSINGS

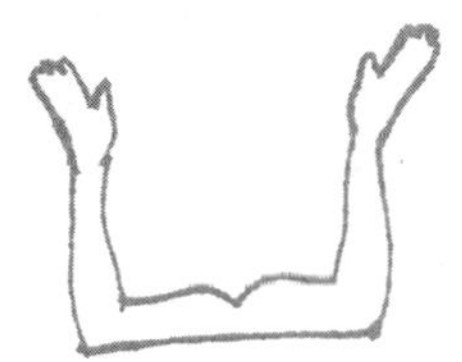

WEEK 2—Blessing the Way: Giving Blessings

The hieroglyph of two raised arms symbolizes the inherent power of goodness in one's soul. The gesture is one of benevolence and can be read as a metaphor for a hug. When we hug someone we pull them toward us and hold them against our heart. We communicate that we want to be at peace with them, and that we wish them well. To hug someone is to bestow a blessing from the goodness of one's heart.

When we are at peace with the other people in our lives we can be at peace with ourselves. The other people in our lives exert a tremendous amount of power over us. Thoughts of them fill our waking and our dreaming life. We become sad, angry, jealous, or depressed by focusing on the faults and shortcomings of others. We dwell on the insensitive way they are treating us or have treated us in the past. We often blame others for why we aren't succeeding or why we can't achieve the happiness we deserve. We feel treated unfairly by others, unloved or not loved enough. We think that we deserve better. We often feel sorry for ourselves and long to be surrounded by loving and supportive people who think we are amazing. Right? And our excuse is always, "If only he would stop . . ." or, "If only she didn't do . . ." We too often feel that other people are in our way—in the way of our happiness. The others in our lives are actually providing us with the way. But we must be willing to see them in that light.

To be free of all the nasty people in your world is possible. Have faith in the knowledge that all the nasty people in your world can change. But don't wait for them to change on their own, or you'll be waiting forever! You must change them yourself. If you want someone to be a holy being, you must see him or her as a holy being. They actually only exist in your own mind anyway. They have come from your own past karmas and appear according to how you see them. How you see anyone or any situation in your present life is due to your past karmas—how you have treated others, in your past. When the great saint Ramana Maharshi was asked, "How should we treat others?" he replied, in yogic fashion, "There are no others." But he was an enlightened being, and enlightened beings live in a reality of oneness. In that state of unitive consciousness, otherness does not exist. Such enlightened yogis do not live in a dualistic reality like most of us do. They see others as their own enlightened Self. If we could see others as our own self we would probably treat them more kindly. We would certainly try our best to treat others as we would like to be treated.

We cannot escape our past karmas—the actions we have already done—but we can start now and do our best to plant the kinds of seeds we want to see grow in the future. Cultivating forgiveness, kindness, and friendliness toward others results in spiritual strength. So much suffering comes from seeing ourselves as a victim of others—as a repository for their selfishness, cruelty, greed, insensitivity, and so forth. We see the world as "out there," coming at us, instead of taking responsibility and realizing that the world we see outside of us has come from *inside* us, from how we have treated others in our past. Others provide us with a karmic projection—a mirror in which to see ourselves.

The way of the yogi is to dive deeper within, past the karmic level to the eternal soul, the unchanging *atman*, which is our connection to God. The nature of the eternal soul is joy, and this is the only true reality; everything else is temporary. When one realizes the nature of his or her own soul they discover the true Self—that which can never be harmed by anyone, that which is *satchidananda* (eternal truth, consciousness, and bliss). Through the practice of giving blessings to others you come closer to the experience of the power of your own soul—the power of goodness.

It is a well-known fact that only saints give blessings. Well, how do you think a saint becomes a saint? Yes, it is through the practice of giving blessings. As the blessing comes through you, it changes you. By giving blessings to someone else you change the negative perception of that person in your own mind and you also change the perception of yourself as someone who sees negativity. Giving blessings is an anonymous way of changing your world—it can turn devils into angels. And it can all happen in the privacy of your own mind—you don't have to "meet them for coffee" and talk it out. If you aren't willing to see someone as a good person, how can you expect him or her to be one? The power is in your hands—well, actually, your mind. The question is, how willing are you to forgive, to let go, and to allow love to lead the way?

Compassion is infinite; you won't run out, so don't be stingy with your blessings—give your blessings to everyone—to the people you don't like as well as the ones you do like. Blessing the ones you love and seeing them as holy beings ensures that they will remain holy, blessed beings in your life.

THE PRACTICE

Allow the image of someone you know to arise in your mind. As you inhale, silently say, "Blessings and love to—" and as you exhale, silently say the name of that person. Continue focusing on that same person or allow other people to float into your consciousness. As you give the blessing try to visualize the person filled with joy and surrounded by light.

> *Option #1:* Remain lying in bed and, with your eyes closed, give blessings to as many people as you feel is right before getting out of bed.
>
> *Option #2:* Sitting comfortably in a meditative posture, use a mechanical timer to keep track of the time, allowing you to focus on giving blessings without worrying about how much time you have. Set the timer and sit

quietly, giving blessings for five to ten minutes or for however long you feel comfortable doing so.

Option #3 (more mystical): Use a *mala* (prayer beads). Hold the mala with your right hand and, while touching each bead with your thumb and ring finger, focus on a person and give the blessing as above. Decide beforehand how many rounds you will go on the mala.

• WEEK 3 •

NOURISHING THE WAY

FEEDING THE BIRDS

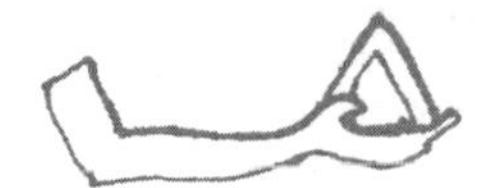

WEEK 3—Nourishing the Way: Feeding the Birds

The hieroglyph of an outstretched arm holding an offering—a wedge of cake or piece of bread in the palm of the hand—represented to the Egyptians charity, the act of sharing nourishing, good food. The secret to wealth is to give generously to others. Whatever we give will come back to us many times over.

Remembering God and being kind to others is the most important job that any of us has in this life. Being kind to others is the essential ingredient to being able to remember God to be able to see ultimate reality. Developing kindness and compassion toward others is the sure way to happiness. But how does that work?, you might ask: Doesn't being kind to others in a charitable way only benefit the others? No. Kindness benefits both the other and yourself. Others do not exist independently; they have come from your past karmas. They only exist in your life because you see them as existing. The Hindu sage Patanjali explains this in the *Yoga Sutras: vastu-samye chitta-bhedat tayor vibhaktah panthah PYS IV.15*. This can be translated to mean: each individual person perceives the same object in a different way, according to their own state of mind and projections. Everything is empty from its own side and appears to you according to how you see it.

When you are unkind to someone, you plant a seed to see unkindness. For example, you judge someone as a greedy person. As soon as you think or say that, you plant a seed that will ensure that greedy people will appear in your life.

When you see yourself as poor, as not having enough to be able to share and be generous to others, you plant seeds for seeing yourself as a victim of poverty, and that will become your reality as you continue to nourish that perception of yourself. You have a choice: you can see yourself as an enlightened being or as a victim, but you can't have both. If you eventually want to see yourself as an enlightened being, then begin that process by seeing others as holy beings. How you treat others will determine how others treat you; how others treat you will determine how you see yourself; how you see yourself will determine who you are.

If you want to rid the world of greed, you must destroy the seeds in your own mind that cause greed to appear in the world. In other words, you must do your best to be kind to others—to take care of others as if they were your own self. Other-centeredness is the secret to overcoming the disease of self-centeredness. Put others before yourself. Be more concerned for the happiness of others than for your own happiness. This will dissolve otherness and reveal the oneness of being. Kindness is the key to Yoga.

Without the development of kindness toward others, you cannot make progress in yoga. Taking care of others is a sure way to increase your own happiness. When we do things with the intention, first and foremost, of making ourselves happy, we only increase our identification with our small self—our body, mind, and personality. In the *Yoga Sutras*, Patanjali cites this identification as the major obstacle to Yoga, calling it *avidya*, which means ignorance or mistaken identity. The yoga practices are designed to help you drop your self-centered concerns and become more other-centered. Being more other-centered expands your sense of self and increases true self-confidence. If you observe unhappy and depressed people you will find that they usually are self-obsessed. The key to uplifting yourself is to do what you can to uplift the lives of others.

Why birds? When you feed the wild birds, you karmically assure that you will always have enough to eat and that wildness will not die inside you. Birds as well as other wild animals are having a hard time surviving in a world dominated by self-centered human beings. When you nourish wildness in another you keep it alive within yourself. Most people assume that birds, being wild, know how to take care of themselves, and feel that taking care of them should not be our responsibility. But the fact is, we have polluted with pesticides or destroyed most of the wild forests and fields where they might have been able to find an abundance of nourishing food. Birds require so little to live—a few good organic seeds and a couple of drops of fresh water—and while it may not be much, it can mean the difference between life and death for a feathered person.

THE PRACTICE

Before you feed yourself—even before you drink a cup of coffee or tea in the morning—feed the birds.

> *Option #1:* Fill up a bird feeder outside your window or at least put some organic seeds or bread crumbs on a windowsill.
>
> *Option #2:* If wild birds aren't nearby, feed your cat, dog, or other family member.

• WEEK 4 •

CONNECTING TO THE WAY

ASANA

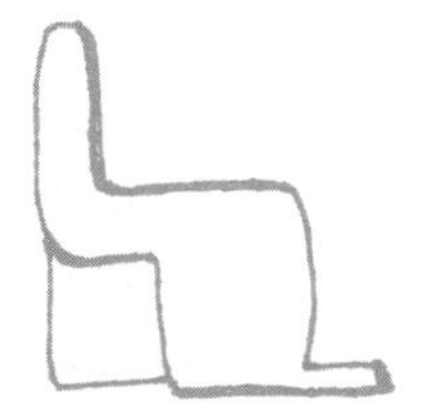

WEEK 4—Connecting to the Way: Asana

The Sanskrit word *asana* means "seat." A seat is a connection to the Earth, implying a relationship. The Egyptian hieroglyph representing the goddess Isis is a seat, an abstract chair, and its phonetic sound is *st*, like the Sanskrit root word *sthit*, which means "stability" (the English word "steady" is related). The ancient Egyptians worshipped the quality of steady connectedness in relationship to the Earth that their goddess Isis embodied. To them she personified the ability to connect perfectly in a relationship. It was Isis who, through the power of love, was able to reassemble the dismembered body of her husband, Osiris, and bring him back to life. She was able to do that because she remembered goodness—the goodness of her eternal soul and the soul's power of love.

Asana practice can bring us to Yoga by helping to purify our relationship to the Earth and all beings. Patanjali in the *Yoga Sutras* says that our asana—our seat, our connection to the Earth—should be *sthira* (steady) and *sukham* (joyful). Our relationship to the Earth should be mutually beneficial—it should benefit ourselves and others. Our lives should not be lived selfishly. If we desire Yoga—to remember our connection to the Supreme Self—everything we do, including our yoga practice, must be done selflessly, with the conscious intention to let go of negative tendencies that urge us to hurt others and to see ourselves as victims. Selfishness disconnects us from the yogi's way.

Is asana a physical or a spiritual practice? To practice yoga you must have a physical body. Your intention while you are practicing asana will determine the result of the practice, and your thoughts are the most powerful force working upon you. For an asana practice to be a spiritual practice the practitioner has to intend it to be. Many people choose to practice yoga asanas only to improve their level of physical fitness, and there is nothing wrong with that. But for those who want more, asana has more to offer. The practice can bring you to enlightenment. How? By helping to shift your perception of yourself and others. Asana can be a therapeutic practice that improves our relationships.

Karma means action. We act in relation to others; everything we think, say, and do involves us with others—other people, animals, trees, plants, and the overall environment. Even our relationship with ourselves is affected by our relationships with others. How we perceive ourselves is dependent upon our relationship with others. Others can hurt our feelings. If we feel that someone we admire doesn't like us, we may worry and start to think that we are somehow flawed. Whereas, experiencing support and encouragement from others can give us confidence and make us feel invincible. It is natural to want to be respected and loved. Relationships that are one-sided are not considered good relationships. If we want to be loved, we must love. If we want to be forgiven, we must forgive. Whatever we want for ourselves we should make happen for others. This consideration must extend to all others and even to the Earth—the environment. To treat others as we want to be treated is the way to establish mutually beneficial relationships, relationships that are steady and joyful. The practice of asana is designed to purify our relationships; it is indeed a very physical practice but with deep emotional and spiritual potential.

The karmas generated by our interactions with others are stored in the tissues of our bodies. In fact, it is our karmas that actually make up our bodies, so moving the body through asana practice, with the intention of purifying our karmas—resolving relationship issues—will help us feel more comfortable in our bodies, resulting in more happiness. When our connection to the Earth and all others is mutually beneficial, we are on our way to Yoga, true Self-realization, the realization of the oneness of being, where otherness disappears.

In Week 4 the focus is asana and we practice the Magic Ten, a series of ten simple asanas that can be done in about ten minutes. The Magic Ten moves the spine in all the various ways that the spine can move. For this reason it is an effective, physically therapeutic daily exercise program that keeps the spine limber and the joints mobile as well as toning muscles and internal organs. The practice will also stimulate the endocrine system, instigating a release of natural, feel-good chemicals such as dopamine. It is akin to accessing your own pharmaceutical laboratory, and the good news is: no negative side effects!

Undertaken with intention, the asana practice can also act as a powerful psychotherapeutic transformational tool with the potential to integrate body, mind, and spirit. The tightness, weakness, and pain that we encounter when doing asanas are physical symptoms hinting at possible deeper emotional causes such as anger, resentment, and blame. For example, if you experience difficulty balancing in a standing asana, like downward facing dog, an unresolved karmic issue with a parent might be indicated. Or if a back-bending asana is hard—as in tabletop, where you need to stretch your chest and open your heart—an inability to forgive someone in your life who has hurt you may be a root cause. Even though it is possible through the practice of asana to heal relationships and move toward enlightened awareness, don't make the mistake of thinking that if someone is really strong and flexible that they must have great relationships and be enlightened. Intention is the deciding factor—what we are thinking about when we do the practice.

Asana, like any other activity, can be done for ego enhancement alone and not contribute at all to more steadiness and joy in our relationships to the Earth and with other beings. That being said, asana practice does have the potential to transform us into kinder people and even move us closer to yogic realization, if we choose to approach it in that way. Because unresolved psychological/karmic issues with others are often held in the body, if we have the patience to place our body into a position, stay there for a time, and breathe consciously while maintaining a positive frame of mind that is free of negativity, we can begin to reconnect with our physical, energetic, emotional, intellectual, and even spiritual selves. This reintegration will result in more peace, calmness, joy, and ease, and less disconnection, stress, worry, and fear. Eventually we may even start to notice an improvement in our relationships with others.

I call it the *Magic* Ten because I think of magic as a shift in perception. After completing the series you will experience your perception of yourself and others in a more optimistic light. You may even begin to see that through connecting to yourself and others in a more positive way there is nothing standing in the way of your achieving happiness—indeed, everything and everyone in your life will provide you with the way.

THE PRACTICE

Before beginning the first asana, mentally state a positive, selfless intention to guide you throughout the series. Here are a few examples:

> "Through this practice may I be able to let go of the toxic physical and emotional poisons that I am holding in my body."
>
> "May this practice help to free me from anger, jealousy, and fear so I can be more loving, forgiving, and kind to others."
>
> "May this practice help me to become an instrument of God's will."
>
> "May this practice help me to enhance the lives of others."
>
> "May this practice shift my perception of myself and others so that I may come to see my enemies as friends, helping me to develop patience and forgiveness."

There are ten exercises in the Magic Ten series. Follow the instructions and breathe evenly, in and out through your nose with your mouth closed and your jaw relaxed, silently counting each breath.

Option (more devotional): Instead of counting the breaths using numbers, insert a mantra. For example, each time you inhale, silently say, "*Hari Om*," and while exhaling count from 1 to 10, or whatever the suggested breath count is.

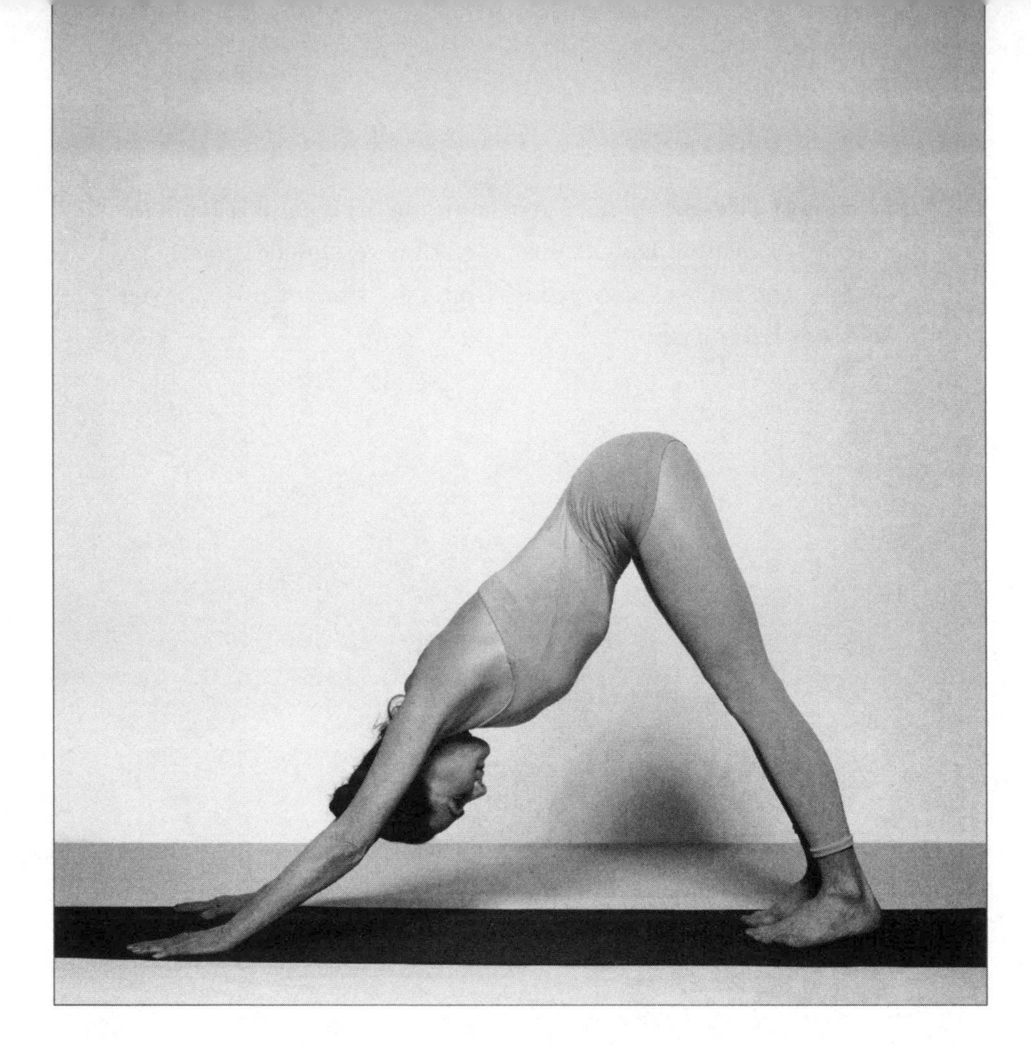

1. DOWNWARD FACING DOG (*ADHO MUKHA SVANASANA*)

Start on your hands and knees. Inhale, lift your knees, exhale while pressing back and up, extending your legs. Reach heels to the floor, release your head, stay, and breathe.

Inhale–Exhale 1 . . . (continue counting through 10 breaths)

Inhale–Exhale 10

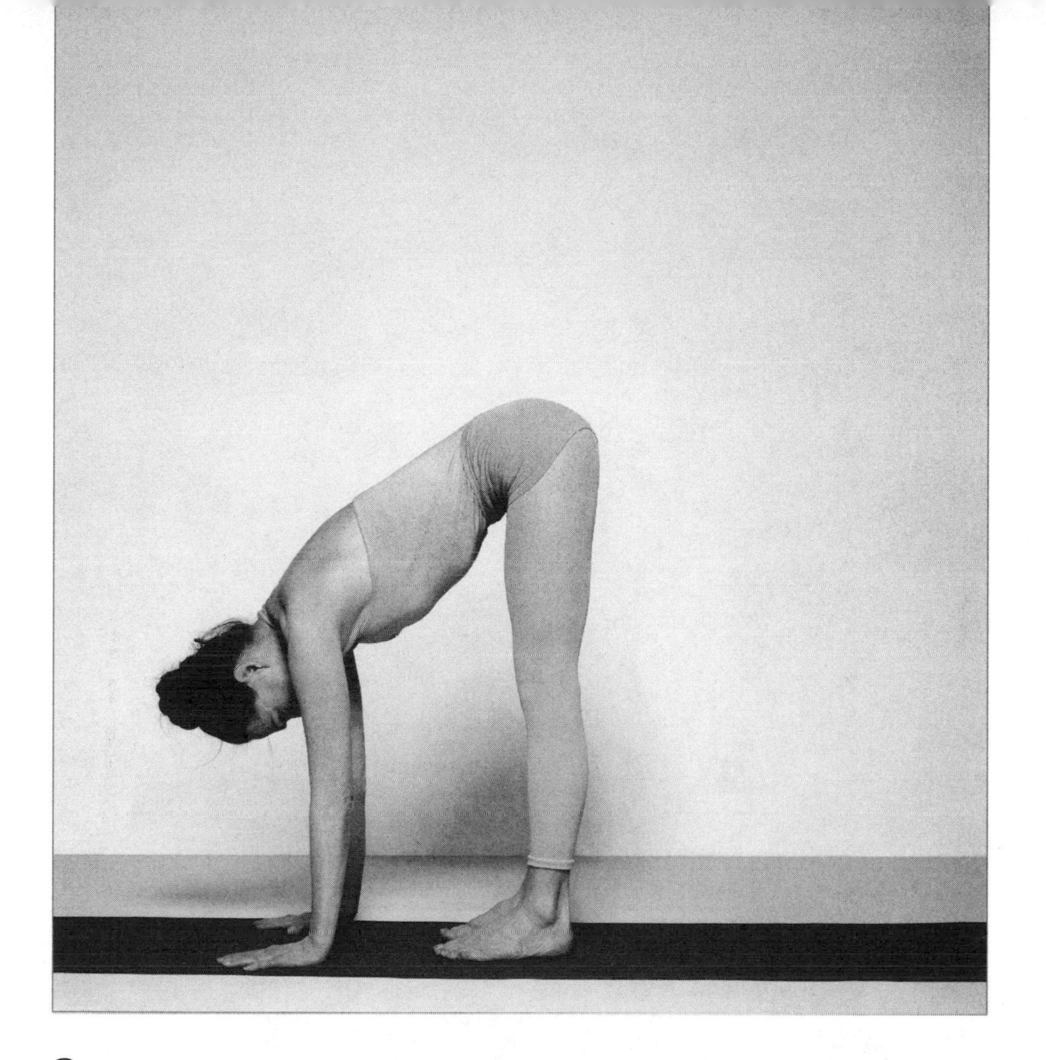

2. STANDING FORWARD BEND (*UTTANASANA*)

Walk the feet forward behind the hands, feet hip-width apart and parallel, palms should be under the shoulders and pressed into the floor. If you can't reach the floor, place each hand on a block—try to keep arms and legs straight. Divide the weight equally between the hands and feet; in other words, don't rock back into the feet or favor one side.

Inhale—Exhale 1 . . . (continue counting through 10 breaths)

Inhale—Exhale 10

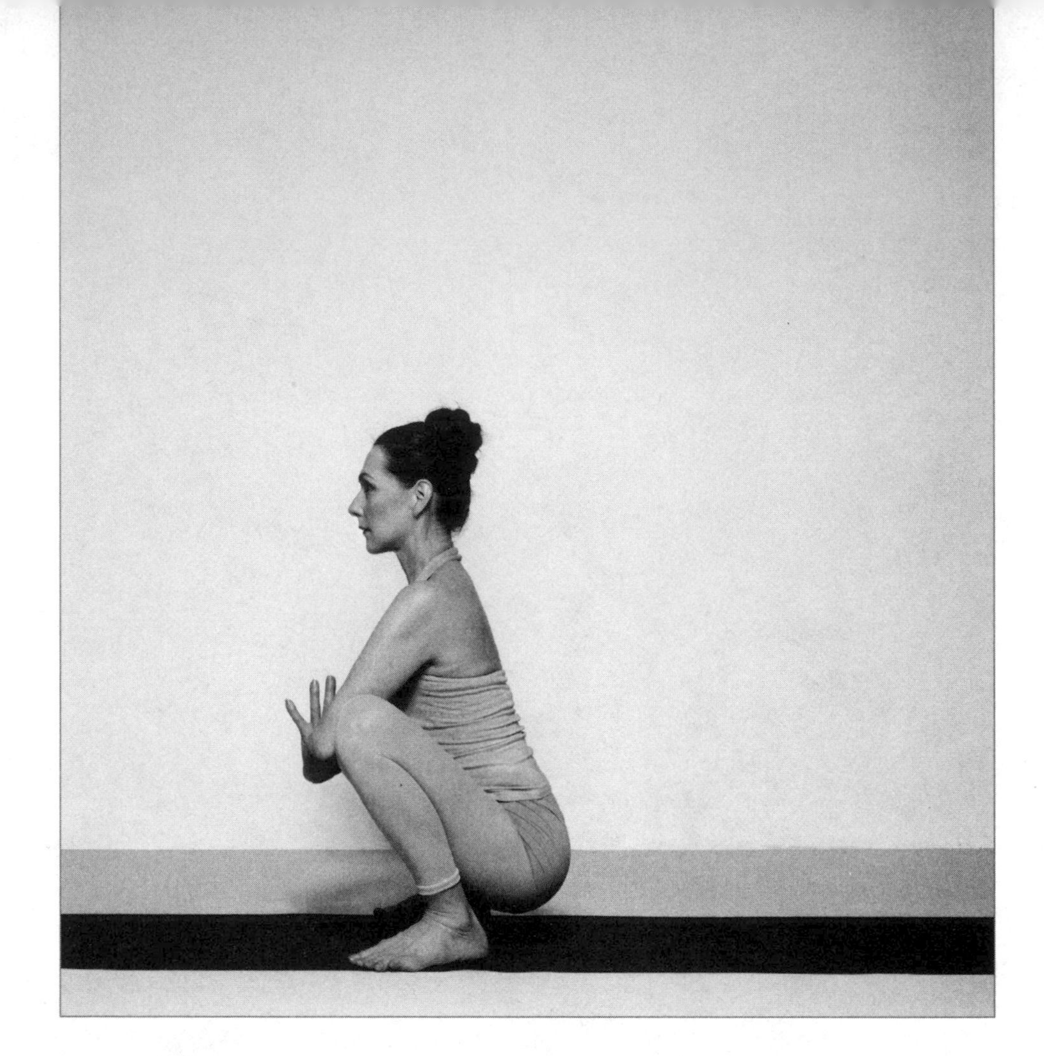

3. SQUAT (*MALASANA*)

Separate the feet mat-width apart, bend the knees to a squatting position, press hands together in prayer, using bent elbows to open the inner thighs, and extend the spine upward. It is acceptable to turn the feet out slightly in order to maintain balance, but make sure the big toe mounds are pressing down and the knees are aligned over the middle of the feet—in other words, be careful not to let your knees roll inward.

Inhale—Exhale 1 . . . (continue counting through 10 breaths)

Inhale—Exhale 10

Option: If you find that your heels don't touch the floor, roll up your mat or insert a blanket under your heels; or sit down on a yoga block.

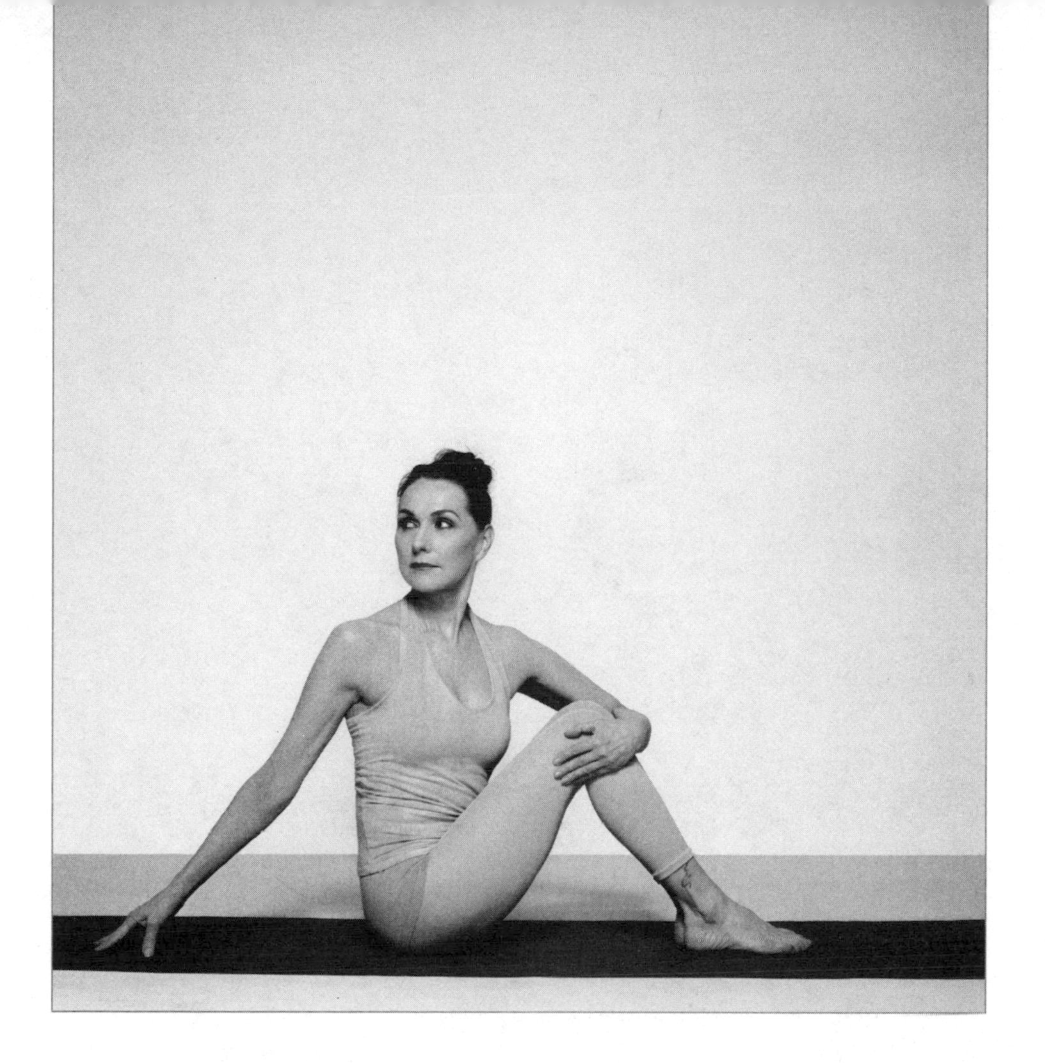

4. TEEPEE TWIST

Sit down and extend both legs forward, then bend your knees, placing the backs of the heels where the backs of your knees were. With knees bent, inner knees and heels touching, wrap your left arm around your shins, place your right hand on the floor behind, and inhale: lengthen your spine, exhale: twist 1 . . . (continue counting through 5 breaths). Inhale: face forward, then repeat, twisting to the left side.

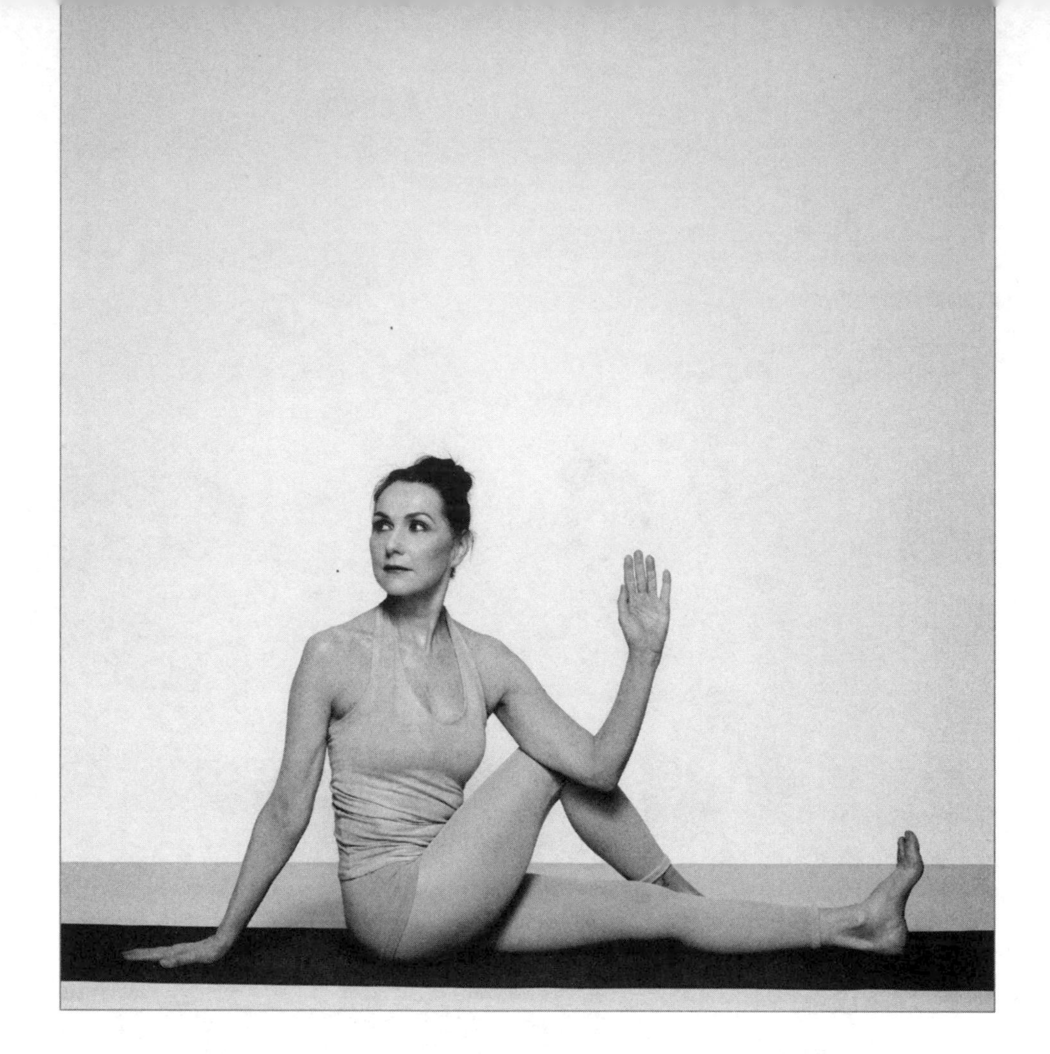

5. HALF-SEATED SPINAL TWIST (*ARDHA MATSYENDRASANA*)

Start with both legs extended on the floor. Inhale, bend the right knee, exhale, place the right foot outside the left calf, placing the right heel on the floor next to the left knee (or move the foot farther down past the knee). Inhale, extend your left arm up, elongating the left side, then exhale, twist to the right, pressing the outside of your left arm against the outside of your right knee, keep the left arm bent at the elbow or hold the right instep with the left hand. Count 5 breaths, then straighten both legs and repeat, twisting to the left side.

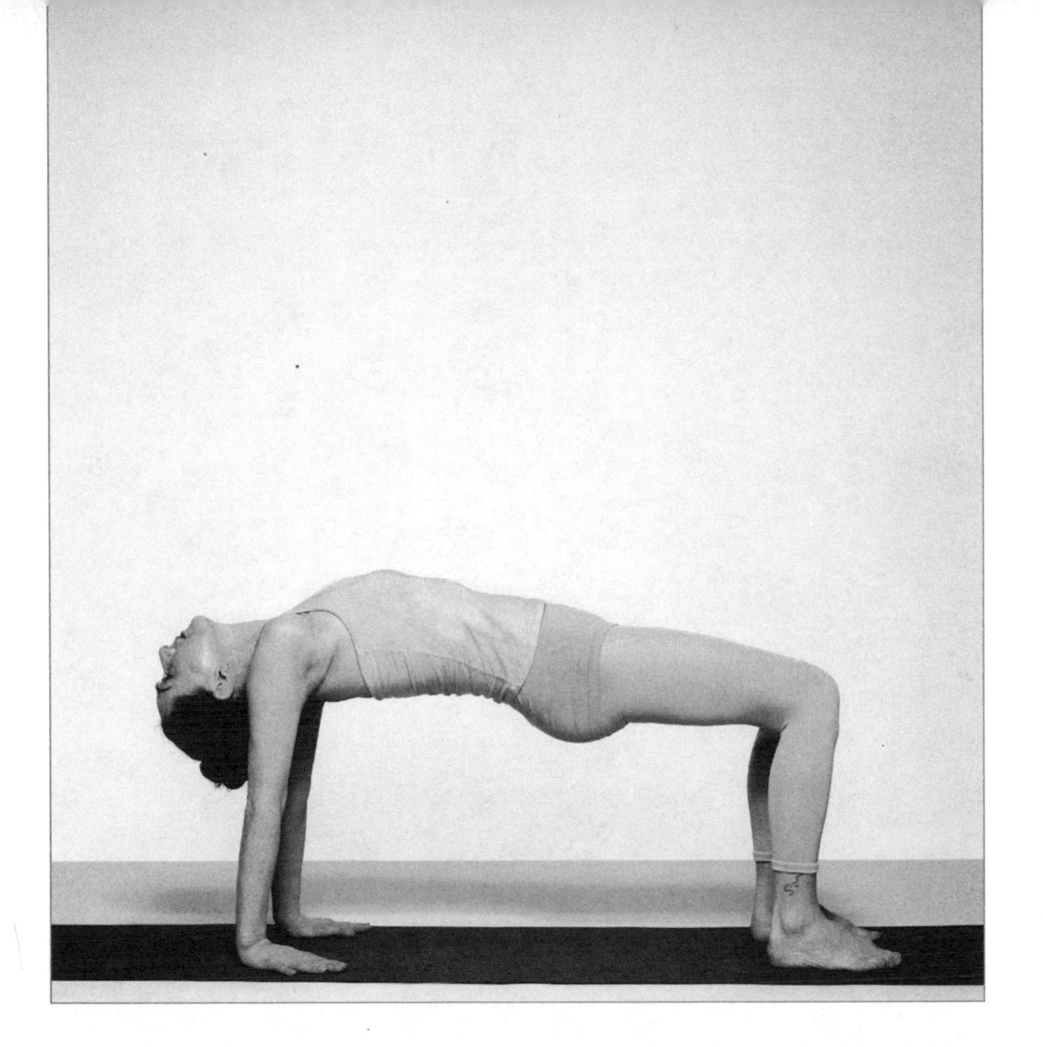

6. TABLETOP

Inhale: bend the knees, place your feet hip-width and parallel, exhale: place hands behind back, fingers facing forward. Inhale, lift pelvis high, exhaling extend the head back. The feet should end up hip-width apart and parallel, with the ankles directly under the knees. The hands should be directly under the shoulders. By pressing the heels down firmly you can continue to keep the pelvis lifted high.

Inhale—Exhale 1 . . . (continue counting through 10 breaths)

Inhale—Exhale 10 and come down

Option (easier): Stop here at the Magic Six, and don't complete the next four asanas.

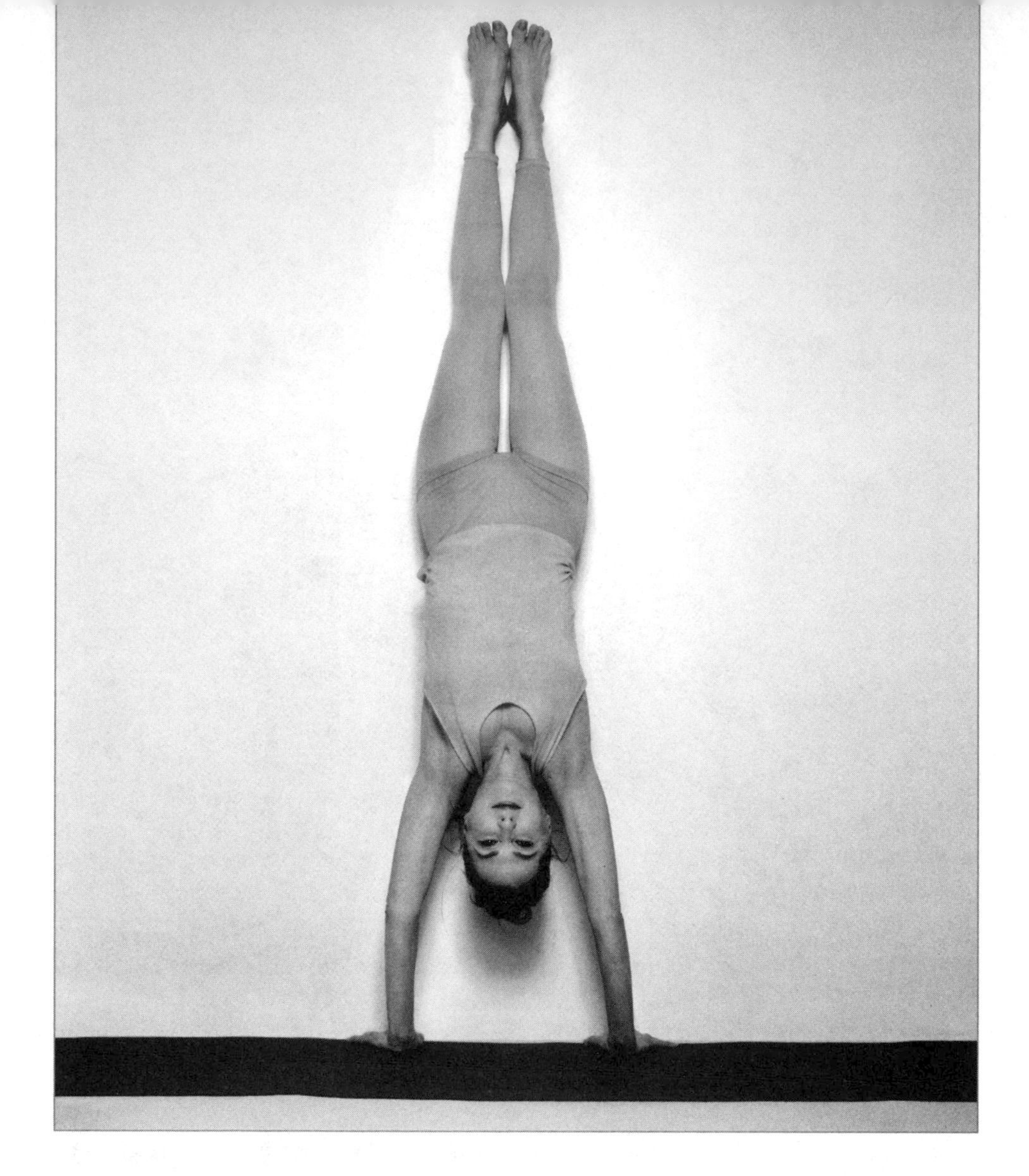

7. HANDSTAND (*ADHO MUKHA VRKSASANA*)

Place your hands palms-down on the floor, and with the tip of your middle fingers about five inches from the wall, walk your feet away until you are in a short downward dog. Then lift one leg, bend the other leg, and kick up into handstand, resting both heels on the wall, and drop your head, keeping the back of your neck long and relaxed. Keep heels on the wall, pressing upward through the balls of your feet while counting breaths. (Start with holding for 5 breaths, then gradually over time—

weeks, months, or years—increase to 50 or more breaths.) Do your best to breathe slow, even breaths in and out through your nose, keeping your mouth closed and your jaw relaxed. Now exhale, come down and, hanging over your legs in a standing forward bend, stay for 2–3 slow breaths, then while inhaling, bend your knees and slowly roll up to standing.

Option (easier alternative version: the L-shaped handstand): Start on the floor on hands and knees, with feet flexed under and heels touching the wall. Make sure your hands are placed in line under your shoulders and your knees are in line under your hips. Lift knees off the floor and walk one foot up the wall, then the other, until both feet are on the wall, with the knees bent. Then straighten both legs as best you can so that the legs are at a 90-degree angle with the torso, making an "L" shape. Drop your head, lengthening your neck. Don't let your weight settle into your wrists; instead, consciously lift the energy up through your arms and out of your wrists, press the heels and balls of feet into the wall, relaxing your toes. Count 5–10 breaths.

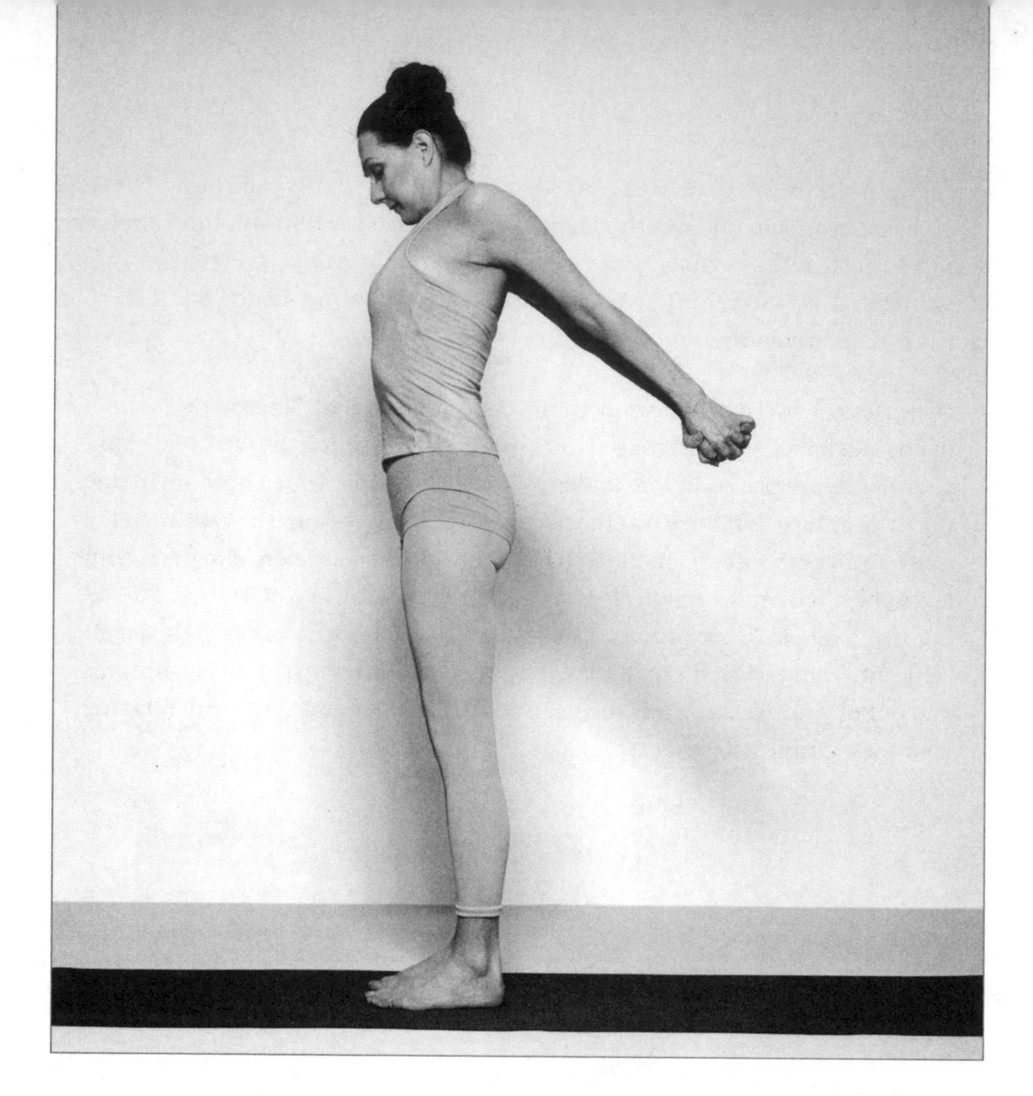

8. CHEST EXPANSION

Stand straight with feet parallel, interlace fingers behind your back, press palms together. Inhale: puff up the chest, drop chin to chest, and lift the arms up and away from the torso. Keep your spine extended and don't tilt your pelvis. Exhale.

Inhale 1 (continue counting through 5 breaths)

Then release hands and arms by the sides of the body.

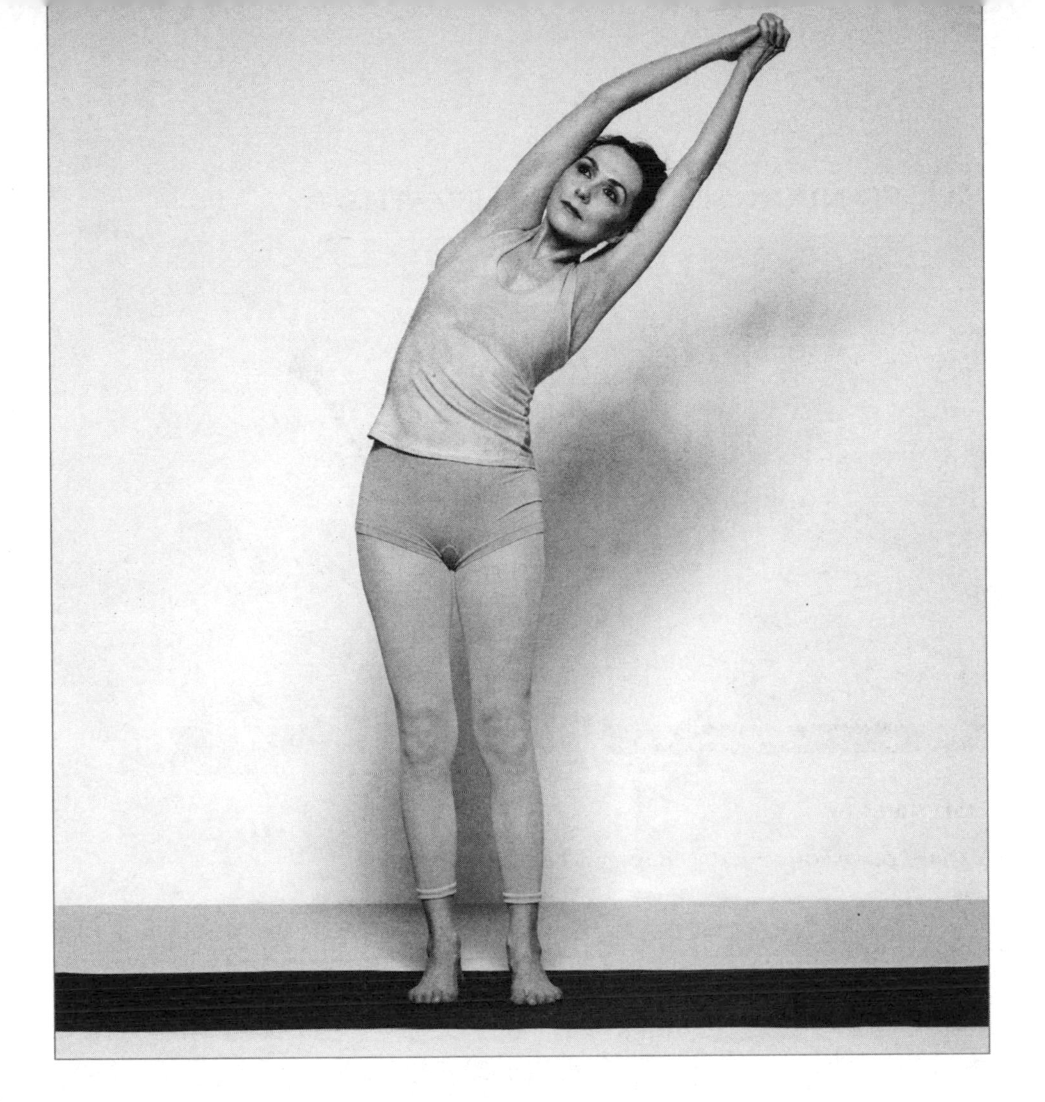

9. SIDE BENDING

Inhale: extend arms over head, interlacing your fingers, palms pressing, relax your shoulders

Exhale: bend to the left (1)

Inhale: back to center

Exhale: bend to the right (2)

Repeat back and forth for 10 bends (a total of 5 on each side)

Option: Instead of 10 bends, do 4 bends (for a total of 2 on each side)

10. STANDING SPINAL ROLL (16 BREATHS)

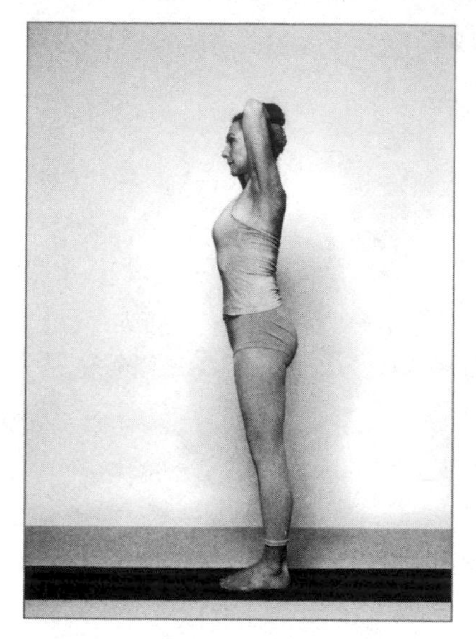

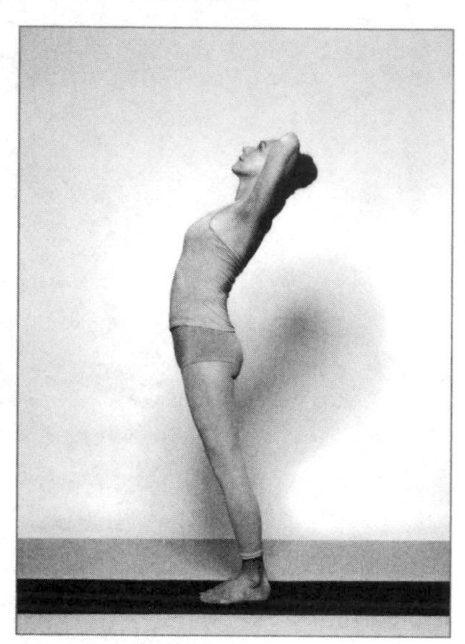

Start standing.

Exhale: place your interlaced fingers behind your head

Inhale: spread elbows, lengthen spine, expand chest

Exhale: arch back (1)

Inhale: lengthen spine

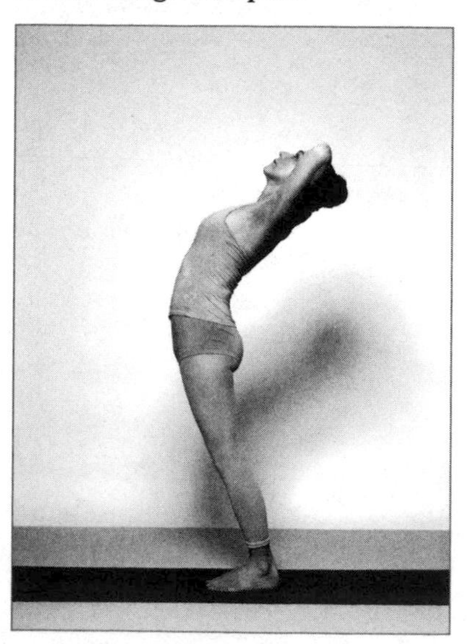

Exhale: lean back farther (2)

Inhale: lengthen spine

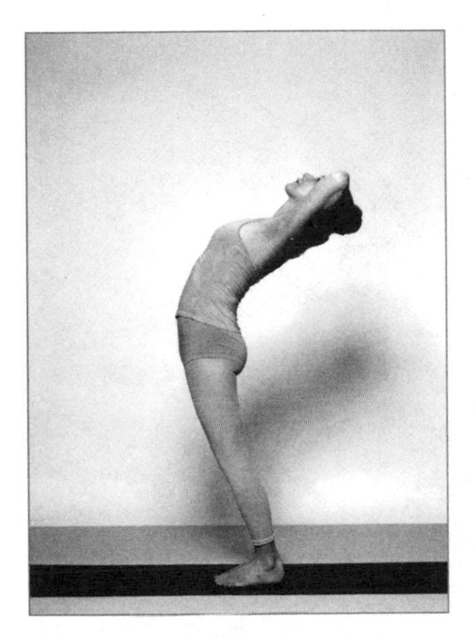

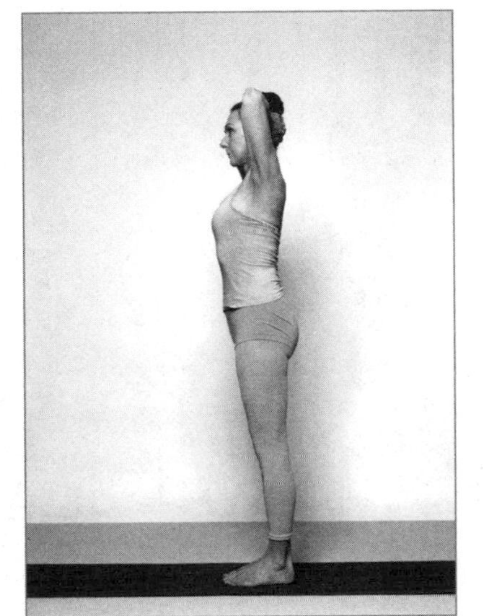

Exhale: lean back farther (3)

Inhale: come to an upright position

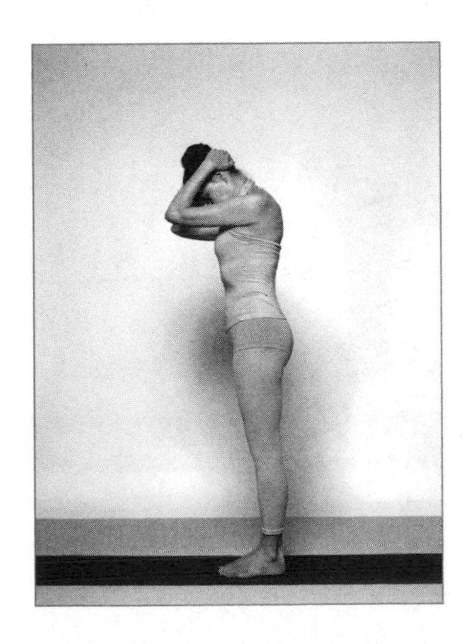

Exhale: draw elbows toward each other, chin to chest (4)

Inhale: bring a sense of expansiveness into the upper back

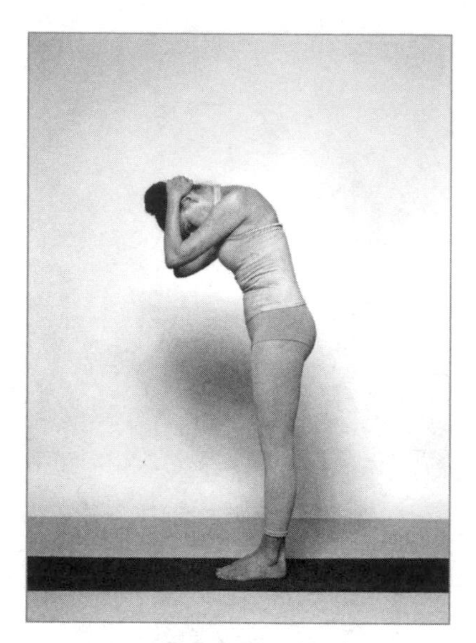

Exhale: roll down nose toward upper chest (5)

Inhale

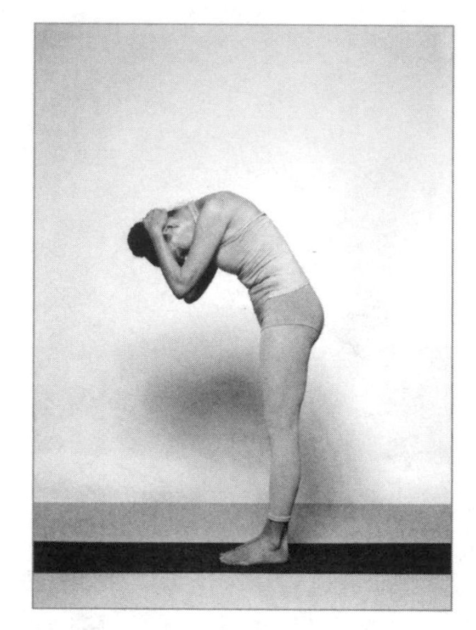

Exhale: roll down forehead toward sternum (6)

Inhale

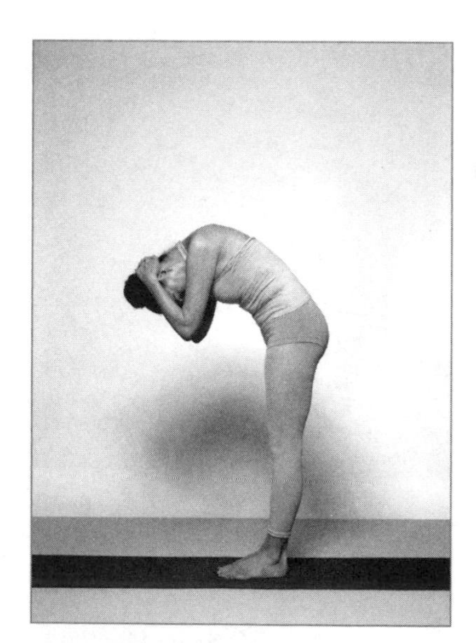

Exhale: roll down forehead toward belly (7)

Inhale

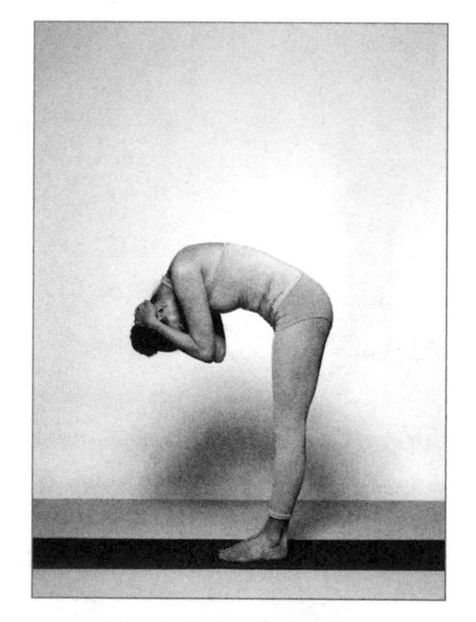

Exhale: roll down forehead toward navel (8)

Inhale

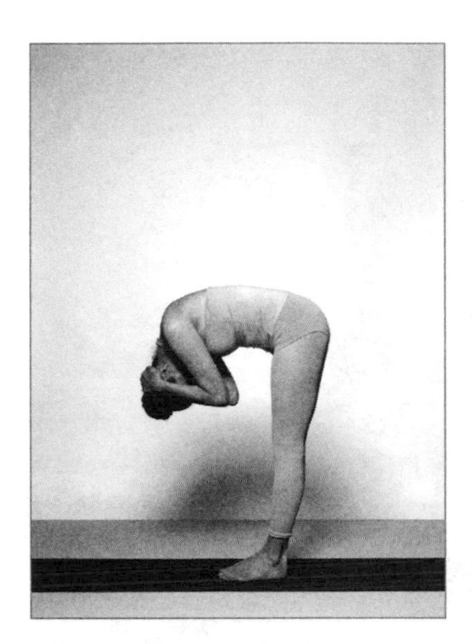

Exhale: roll down forehead toward pubic bone (9)

Inhale

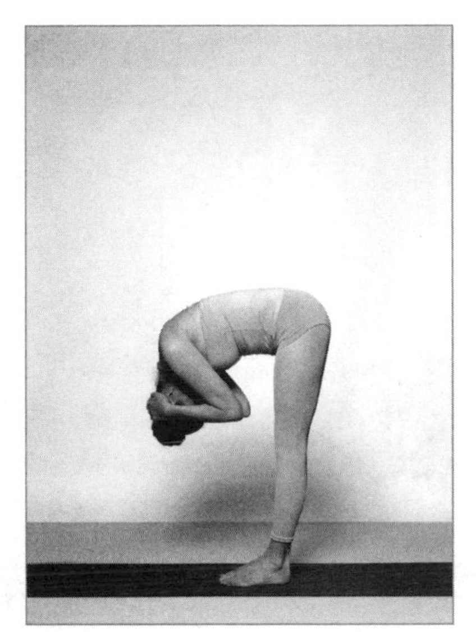

Exhale: roll down forehead to mid thighs (10)

Inhale

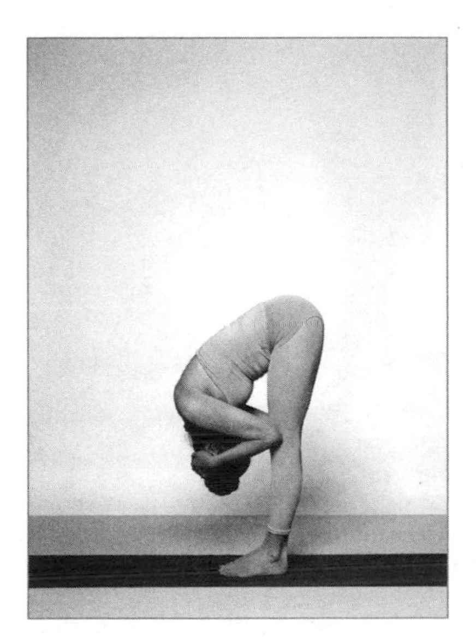

Exhale: roll down forehead toward knees (11)

Inhale

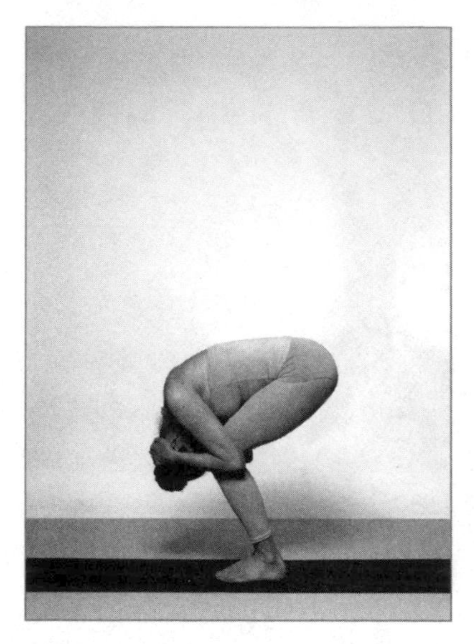

Exhale: bend knees, touching forehead to knees, elbows touching outside of knees (12)

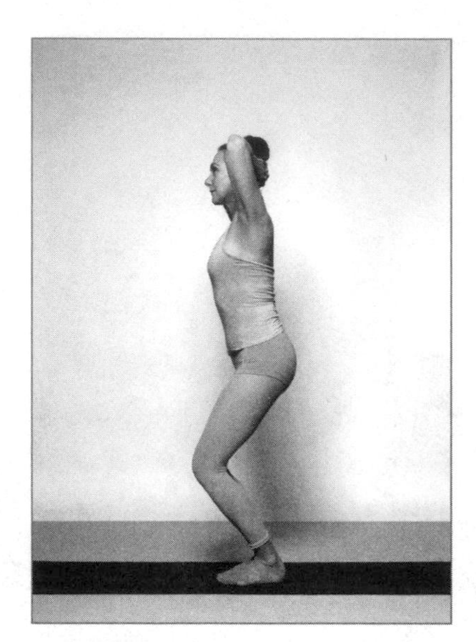

Inhale: keep knees bent, open elbows, lift torso, maintain a straight spine

Exhale: stay (13)

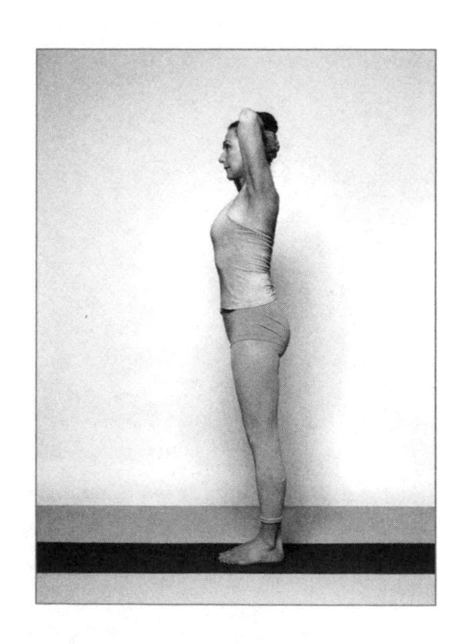

Inhale: straighten legs, lift to upright position

Exhale: (14)

Inhale: lengthen spine

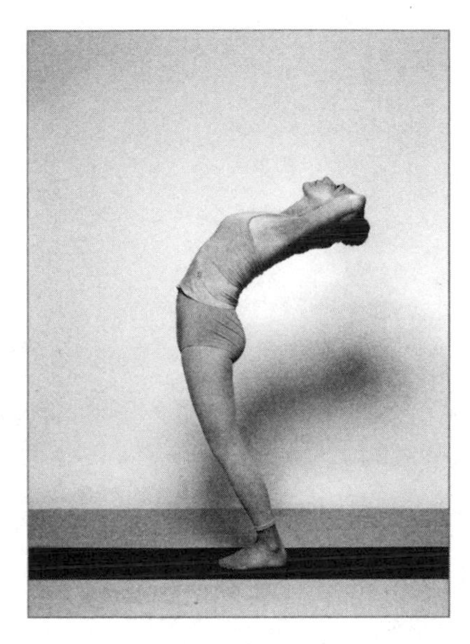

Exhale: lean back as far as is comfortable (15)

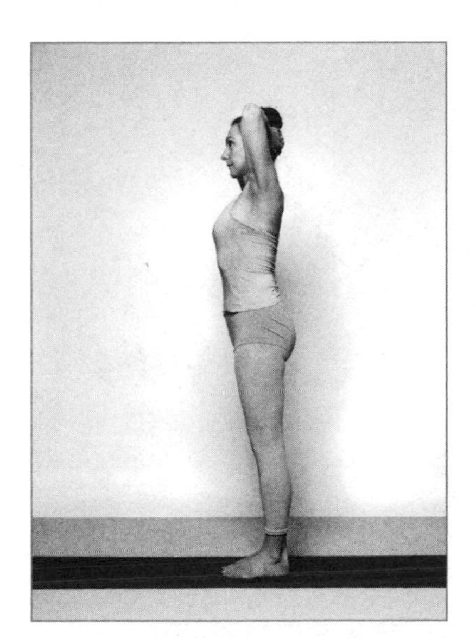

Inhale: come to upright position

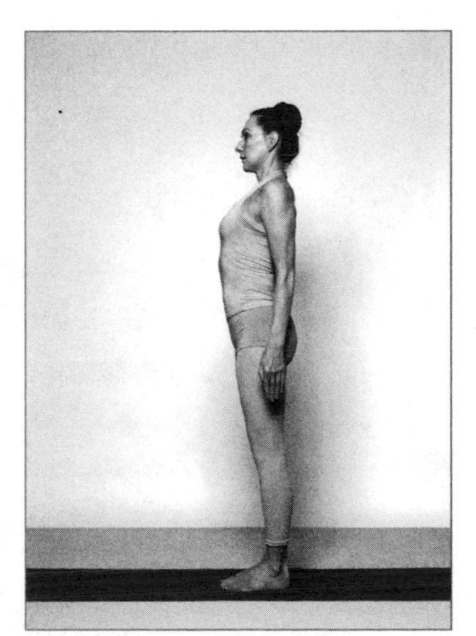

Exhale: release arms to sides (16)

Option (easier)*:* Don't try to keep the legs straight during breaths 5–12, instead soften the knees as you roll down.

• WEEK 5 •

MOVING THROUGH THE WAY

DANCE

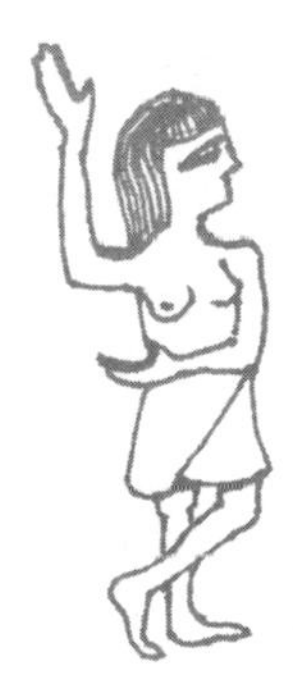

WEEK 5—Moving Through the Way: Dance

The earliest archaeological evidence for early dance has been found in two places, India and Egypt. In ancient Egypt dance was a part of life, played an important role in the lives of all social classes, and was performed both publicly and privately as a way to express, through music and movement, a connection to the spiritual vibrational realm—that which cannot be seen but can be felt. Music is like air—it is everywhere. To dance is to tap into the eternal presence of music, allowing it to move through your body. The lives of the ancient Egyptians were saturated with religious feeling and they lived close to nature. Their gods communicated to them through the living world around them, in the wind and the reeds blowing by the river and in the movements of the birds across the sky and the snake slithering on the surface of the sand. Dancers danced solo, in pairs, or in groups. In pair dancing it was always two men or two women; women and men did not dance together socially as is our custom today.

Dancing by yourself is a joyful experience that looses inhibitions, develops musicality, and increases joy. The three steps that form this basic routine are quite invigorating. Some people may recognize these movements from the respected American tradition of aerobics popular during the 1980s.

THE PRACTICE

The three simple dance movements stimulate the cardiovascular system—accelerating heart rate and increasing blood circulation—and improve physical coordination, increase joy, and gracefully teach us how to synchronize breath with movement.

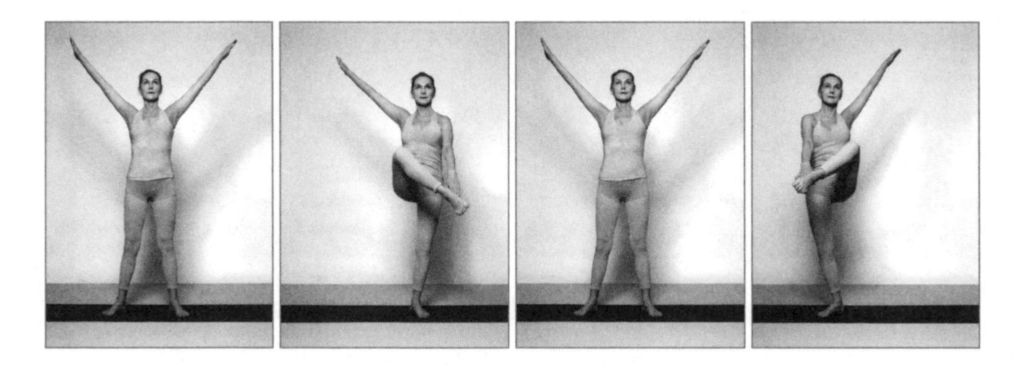

Start out standing with legs open and both arms stretched and lifted above head, your body forming an X shape.

Leg lifts to the front 10 breaths. Lift your right leg, bending the knee, turning it out at the hip so that the inside of your leg is facing upward, and touch your inner right heel with your left hand. Keep your right arm lifted high, then repeat with the other foot and arm. Go back and forth 10 times, exhaling each time you touch your hand to your heel. Inhale in between lifts when your foot is released to the floor and both your arms are lifted high.

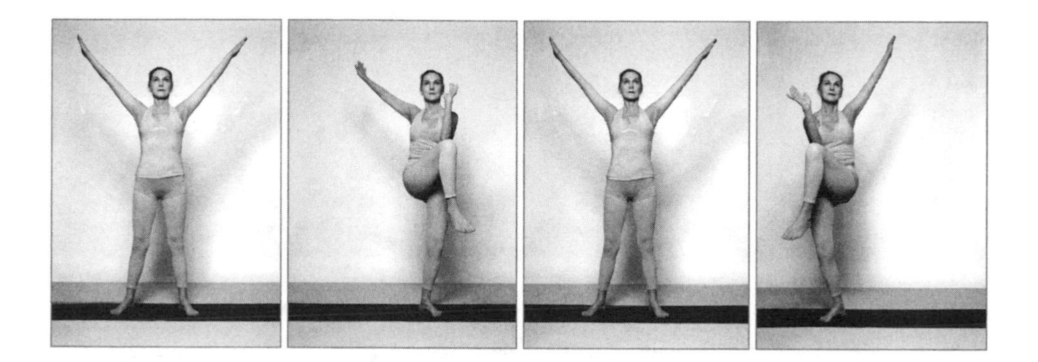

Leg lifts twist 10 breaths. Bend your right knee and lift it high to the front and across the body to the left as you twist, then exhale, bending the left elbow and pressing the outside of the left elbow against the outside of the right knee, or as close as you can come. Then repeat, starting with the other leg. Go back and forth 10 times. Inhale in between lifts every time the foot is released to the floor and both arms are lifted high.

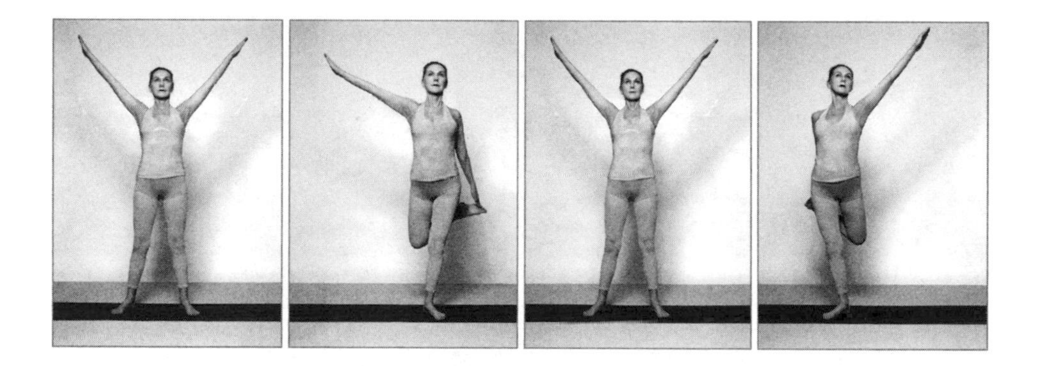

Leg lifts to the back 10 breaths. Bend your right knee and lift your right foot to the back, reach down with your left hand and touch your right heel, then repeat with the other foot and arm. Go back and forth 10 times. Exhale every time you touch your heel with your hand. Inhale in between lifts when the foot is released to the floor and both arms are lifted high.

• WEEK 6 •

SWEEPING THE WAY

KRIYAS

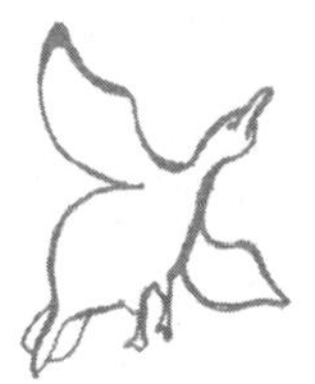

WEEK 6—Sweeping the Way: Kriyas

The bird flies upward, away from all that might be pulling her downward into unnecessary activities and concerns unrelated to her true purpose—remembering God and being kind to others.

In Week 6 we begin the *kriyas*, or cleansing exercises, from the traditional Hatha Yoga system. The following two exercises focus on the basics involved in regulating the *prana*, or life force. They help to sweep clean the subtle energetic channels.

In the Yogic tradition it is said that there are 72,000 energetic channels or conduits called *nadis* running through the astral body, connecting the subtle body with the physical body. Through this network of invisible channels, prana, or the life force, flows. Prana circulates in five directions in the body. These five "winds" of prana are called *vayus*, and they perform different functions: *prana* vayu moves from the diaphragm to the base of the throat and regulates heartbeat, blood circulation, and speech; *apana* vayu flows downward from the navel to the feet and controls urination, defecation, menstrual flow, birth, and ejaculation; *samana* vayu occupies the space around the navel, where it flows back and forth like a pendulum, regulating digestion; *udana* vayu flows from the base of the throat to the top of the head and regulates swallowing as well as coughing, choking, and hiccupping; and *vyana* vayu flows in all directions, carrying prana to every cell of the body.

The practice of *bandhas*—energetic locks—along with kriyas and *pranayama* sweep the subtle wind channels clean. *Uddiyana bandha* is activated only on an exhaled retention. The entire abdomen is lifted inward and upward toward the chest cavity, hence the name, "flying-up," which is what the Sanskrit word *uddiyana* means. It is important to remember than uddiyana is not an abdominal contraction; rather it is a strong lift of the diaphragm muscle, creating a powerful internal vacuum that pulls the abdomen muscles inward and upward. If done correctly the diaphragm muscle will lift high enough to embrace the heart. Because the diaphragm and heart are making such intimate contact, circulation is enhanced and the heart is strengthened.

When the pumping action of *agni sara*, or fire washing, is added after uddiyana bandha the internal organs get squeezed and massaged by the diaphragm muscle, helping to keep them fit and free of toxins. Both of the practices described here (uddiyana bandha and agni sara) create a feeling of renunciation—of thinning out—letting go of things that don't contribute to increasing one's *bhava*, the devotional unitive mood that promotes the remembrance of God and kindness toward others—essential to the yogi's way.

THE PRACTICE

Flying-up Lock (*Uddiyana Bandha*)

Start standing, with your legs apart and a bit wider than your hips and feet parallel or slightly turned out. Inhale a full breath through your nose while expanding the chest and slightly arching the back. As you exhale through your mouth, bend the knees, rest the palms of the hands on the thighs, straighten the arms, and strongly lift the diaphragm muscle up and under the ribs, which will create an internal vacuum that draws the abdomen inward and upward. Tuck the chin toward the chest, keep the lumbar spine long, and close your eyes, gently gazing upward. Hold the exhale retention for a silent count of 10, then stand up straight, release the chin and inhale, causing the diaphragm to move downward. That is 1 round. Repeat for a total of 3 rounds.

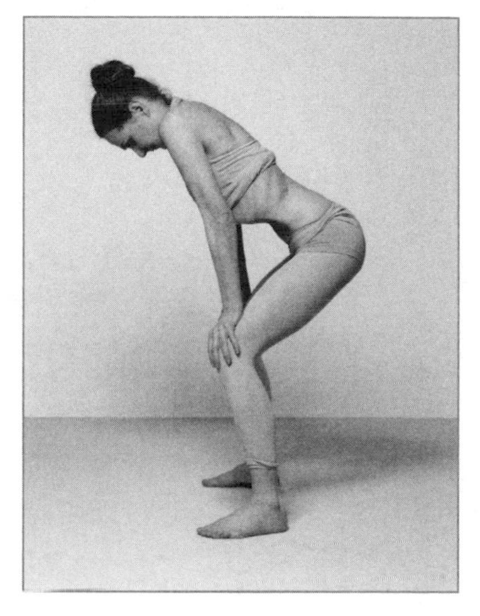

Fire Wash (*Agni Sara*)

Start standing. Follow the instructions for uddiyana bandha, but instead of holding for a count of 10, pump the abdomen by lifting and lowering the diaphragm muscle 10 times to complete 1 round. Repeat for 3 rounds. While you are pumping, the breath should be held out—in other words, don't breathe. In between rounds stand up straight, release the chin, and inhale as you would after uddiyana bandha.

• WEEK 7 •

SHINING THE WAY

KAPALABHATI

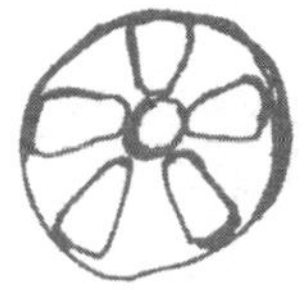

WEEK 7—Shining the Way: Kapalabhati

The hieroglyph of a star inside a circle is the symbol for the soul that shines eternally in the celestial world. Just as the twinkling stars in the sky can light our way, helping us to navigate and find our way home, our souls are meant to shine like stars and help us find our way back to our true heavenly home. Each of us is destined to be a saint, to exemplify happiness and joy, illuminating the way for ourselves and others.

In Week 7 we continue with another kriya, or cleansing practice, from the traditional Hatha Yoga system called *kapalabhati*, which translated from Sanskrit means "skull shining." *Kapala* means "head" and *bhati* means "to polish." Through regular practice of kapalabhati the mind will be cleansed of negative thoughts. This will result in the aura around your head appearing as a shining halo—like the glow that can be seen radiating from the heads of saints.

The exercise might appear at first to look like a way to clear the nostrils and strengthen the abdomen, but if you want to utilize it as a yogic practice—something to help you diminish your ego, rid you of selfish tendencies, and develop devotion—it can be that, too. Think of each exhale as an offering. To the yogi, the only real dirt is *avidya*, which means ignorance of the true Self. Cleansing practices like kapalabhati have been designed to get rid of dirt, and light the way to the Truth—to bring about an enlightening. Kapalabhati is far from being just a simple physical exercise to release phlegm from the respiratory passages. When seen from a yogic perspective it is actually a devotional practice, which increases *bhakti*, or love for God. How? Each time you exhale you are lifting energy upward, from the solar plexus region, the site of the *manipura* chakra. This is the place where your individual will, or ego, is located. With each strong exhale the diaphragm muscle is actually pulled upward to the heart, where it is able to embrace the heart for a split second. The *anahata* chakra is found in the heart center, the place of love and compassion. Know that wherever you look receives your energy. As you close your physical eyes and maintain your gaze toward the third eye (*ajna* chakra), the place of transcendental wisdom, while you are pumping the energy upward, your head gets brighter. With the practice of kapalabhati, each exhaled breath is an offering of your ego, with all of its ignorance, upward through the heart to the wisdom and joy of the transcendental illumined Self.

THE PRACTICE

Kapalabhati: We will do two versions of this potent practice.

Here's the instruction for the basic practice: Sit comfortably with your spine as extended as possible and your head balanced on top of the spine, chin parallel to the Earth. For how to properly sit, please refer to the next chapter, Week 8, Directing the Way: Pranayama, where you will find various appropriate seated positions explained.

Close your eyes gently. Take a full breath in through both nostrils, then exhale sharply, lifting the diaphragm strongly up. Feel as if you are pushing the air up and out through the nostrils. Continue with strong, slow, sharp exhales, making sure you allow for a passive inhale to occur in between each exhale. Keep your eyes closed throughout the practice, and gaze upward toward the third eye (ajna chakra). Make sure to keep your mouth closed throughout the exercise. Keep your shoulders relaxed; don't allow them to move up and down with each pumping. Maintain a calm, relaxed face throughout—no eyebrow gymnastics!

Do 3 rounds of 10 pumpings (exhales) each round. In between each round, take a few relaxing breaths by inhaling and exhaling slowly through both nostrils.

Option (easier): If doing 10 pumpings is too difficult, start with just 5 pumpings and gradually over weeks or months work up to 10.

Option (more advanced): Increase the number of pumpings from 10 to 20 or 30. But be careful not to hyperventilate; make sure your pumpings are done in an even, rhythmic way and not too fast.

Alternate nostril kapalabhati: This is a variation of the basic practice. This version of the kapalabhati practice purifies and balances the left (*ida*) and right (*pingala*) channels or nadis. Once these channels are balanced, prana can enter into the central (*sushumna*) channel and facilitate the ascending of consciousness (*kundalini*) upward to the higher chakras, or levels of perception.

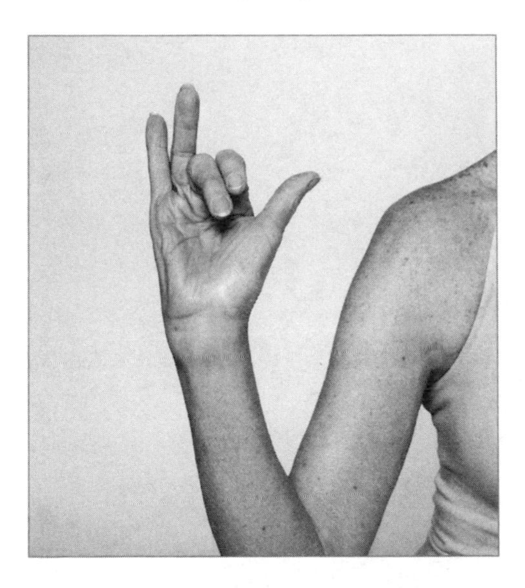

Make *vishnu mudra* with the right hand, by bending the right index and middle fingers down toward the palm, and use the right thumb and ring finger to regulate the breath through the right and left nostrils. Inhale through both nostrils, close right nostril with the right thumb, exhale sharply 11 times through the left nostril, then switch, and using the right ring finger to close the left nostril, exhale sharply 11 times through the right nostril. Switch again, reducing the number of exhales in a descending way, 11-9-7-5-3-1. When you get to 1, exhale sharply 1 breath 11 times back and forth through alternating nostrils. The 11th or last exhale should be through the left nostril. Relax your right hand, bringing it down to rest on your right thigh.

Note: In both of the versions detailed above, make sure that each exhale or pumping is quite strong—a similar feeling to blowing your nose. Allow the inhalation in between exhales to be passive. But also remember to make sure that you *do* inhale in between each exhale, but in a shallow way. Do not make the inhalation as strong as the exhalation; if you do, you may hyperventilate and become dizzy, which is not good.

• WEEK 8 •

DIRECTING THE WAY

PRANAYAMA

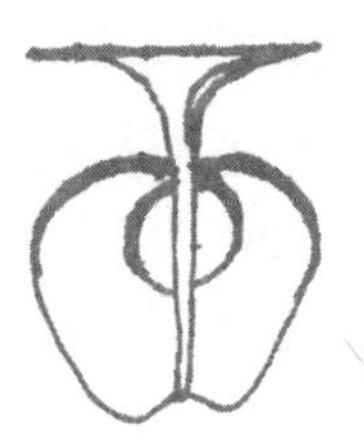

WEEK 8—Directing the Way: Pranayama

The hieroglyph here is an abstract anatomical representation of lungs, heart, and trachea. The image is said to represent a good person, one who lived his or her life perfectly, whose every breath emanated from the deepest place of a pure heart.

In Week 8 we graduate to a traditional pranayama practice from the Hatha Yoga system. *Prana*, as we've seen, is the life force and *yama* means to restrict, control, or regulate. Prana is not the breath, but can be accessed through breathing. Prana is not just present in the external air we breathe, but it is also the internal energetic animating force of life inside every cell of the body. The yogic texts all agree that to be able to consciously regulate the breath is to have control of one's thoughts, and if you are in conscious control of your thoughts you can regulate your life. Through pranayama you make breathing, which to most people is automatic and unconscious, a conscious experience. To become fully conscious is the way of Yoga.

From a physical health perspective, deep-breathing practices like pranayama, which emphasize all four parts of the breath, not only expand our lung capacity but also benefit the kidneys because the urinary and respiratory systems collaborate to help maintain a normal pH or acid–alkaline balance in the blood. This is important for our health because when our pH is out of balance our metabolism—which is our ability to assimilate oxygen as well as derive energy from the food we eat and expel the waste products we need to get rid of—is compromised. This metabolic dysfunction can contribute to many problems, including nervous tension, fatigue, asthma, digestive upsets, constipation, weight gain, and premature aging. The ability to regulate your breathing through pranayama exercises can have a dramatic effect on your overall health. As you continue to practice you will develop more grace and ease and will become more comfortable in your body.

Improving one's diet is the first step to improving one's breathing. Ancient scriptures such as the *Hatha Yoga Pradipika*, in which the techniques of pranayama are explained, caution that before embarking on a regular practice of pranayama, the practitioner should purify his or her diet. According to the yogic dictates, a pure diet is typified by the quality of *sattva*, which means lightness. The food that a yogi consumes should be sattvic—it should not be heavy—and should be easy to digest, resulting in a feeling of lightness. This would naturally point to a pure diet—a vegan diet consisting of organic fruits, vegetables, nuts, and grains. There is no place in a yogi's diet for *tamasic* (heavy) foods like meat and dairy products.

The first thing we do when we come into this world is to inhale, and the last thing we will do upon leaving is to exhale—and in between the time of birth and death is your life. Being able to breathe easily is to be at ease with your life. Pranayama practices help you to develop ease of being—feeling comfortable in your own skin and with whatever comes your way in life.

THE PRACTICE

There are many pranayama practices, but basically they can be divided into the equal or unequal regulation of the breath. We will focus on a practice of equal breathing called *Samavritti Pranayama*. *Sama* means "same," *vritti* means "fluctuations," and so *samavritti* means "same fluctuations" or to balance or equalize the fluctuations. As we said earlier, *pranayama* means directing the life force, so in samavritti pranayama we are directing the life force by evenly regulating the four parts of the breath. The four parts of the breath are: the inhalation (*puraka*), the retention of the inhalation (*antar-kumbhaka*), the exhalation (*rechaka*), and the retention of the exhalation (*bahya-kumbhaka*). To be able to effectively direct the prana, pranayama practice always includes the practice of bandhas.

Bandha means "a lock," as in a pressure regulator. *Mula bandha* (root lock) is the first bandha for the yogi to master. On a general physical level, mula bandha can be described as a contraction of the pelvic floor combined with a strong energetic lift upward. Men can feel this by strongly contracting the space between the anus and genitals. Women can feel mula bandha by contracting the vaginal walls, lifting in and up. *Jalandhara bandha* means "cloud-catching lock." Physically, it consists of lifting the chest so that the chin rests in the depression between the collarbones. *Uddiyana bandha* has already been explained in Week 6; please refer to that chapter for a refresher if you need to. As with any yoga practice, the most exalted application of any bandha is to devote it to enlightenment—where the practitioner becomes fixated or locked on God.

The way you sit to practice pranayama is important, so before focusing on regulating the breath, you need to choose a good seat. Always strive to sit comfortably with a straight spine that is perpendicular to the Earth.

According to the Hatha Yoga tradition, the following cross-legged positions are recommended for both pranayama and meditation practices: *padmasana*, *ardhapadmasana*, *siddhasana*, and *sukasana*. It is helpful, when sitting cross-legged on the floor, to sit on a pillow or folded blanket so that tension does not accumulate in the groin or lower back. Blankets can also be folded and placed under each knee to provide additional support and comfort. The level of the seat should always be higher than the knees.

Padmasana (lotus seat) is done by placing the right foot on top of the left thigh, as close to the pelvis as possible, then lifting the left foot and placing it on top of the right thigh, as close to the pelvis as possible. The soles of both feet should turn upward. To sit in *ardhapadmasana* (half lotus seat), sit cross-legged, placing the right foot on top of the left thigh, then the left foot under the right leg. *Siddhasana* (accomplished seat) is done by pressing the left heel against the perineum, or vaginal opening, and tucking the left toes between the calf and thigh of the right leg, then placing the right heel on top of the left heel and tucking the right toes between the calf and thigh of the left leg. To sit in *sukasana* (easy cross-legged seat), spread a blanket or rug under your buttocks and feet to provide a padded surface and cross your legs at the ankles or shins. Place one or more cushions under your seat so that your knees drop gently toward the floor. If your knees end up hanging in midair, place additional padding underneath each knee.

If you prefer to sit in a parallel kneeling-like position rather than a turned-out cross-legged one, sit in *virasana* or *vajrasana*. To sit in *virasana* (hero seat), first kneel, placing both knees together, then place your hands behind the backs of the knees and pull the skin of the calves down toward the feet and slightly outward. Slowly releasing your hands, sit all the way down, preferably on a cushion, folded blanket, towel, or yoga block. Your feet should be parallel and outside of your hips with the soles facing up. *Vajrasana* (thunderbolt seat) is done by kneeling and sitting on the insides of both your feet, letting one of the big toes overlap the other.

If none of these traditional positions are doable for you, then sit in a chair, but make sure you choose a chair that is not too soft and has a straight back, preferably with no arms. When sitting in a chair do not cross your legs. Keep your legs and feet parallel to each other and make sure your feet touch the floor. If your feet don't touch the floor, put a block, box, or cushion under them. When beginning, go ahead and lean back against the chair, but eventually, as you practice you will gain the strength to sit upright so that your spine is more extended and you won't need the support of the back of the chair.

After you have chosen a seat that works for you and settled into it, breathe a few slow and steady breaths in and out through your nostrils. Now you are ready to start the practice.

After exhaling through both nostrils, apply mula bandha, using vishnu mudra: with the right hand, close the right nostril with the thumb. Inhale through the left nostril for a count of 8 (count silently). Close the left nostril with the ring finger (holding both nostrils closed), and retain the inhaled breath for 8 counts, and additionally apply jalandhara banda. Maintain the bandhas and lift the thumb, exhaling through the right nostril for a count of 8. Close both nostrils and retain the exhaled breath (holding the breath out) for a count of 8. Lift the thumb and inhale into the right nostril for a count of 8, close both nostrils, hold the inhaled breath for 8 counts, lift the ring finger and exhale through the left nostril for a count of 8, close both nostrils, keeping the breath held out for a count of 8. That is the end of the first round. Continue for 7 rounds.

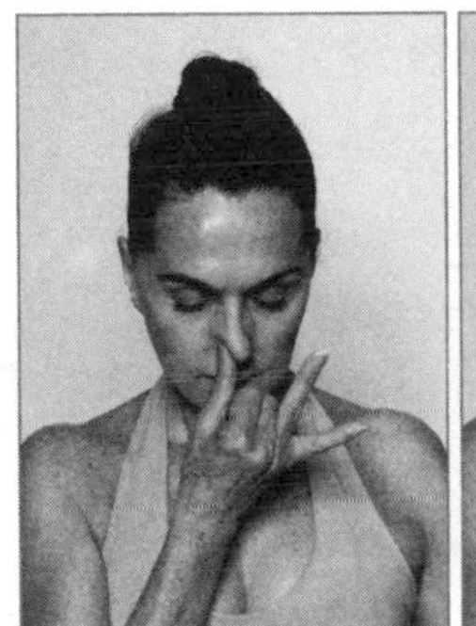
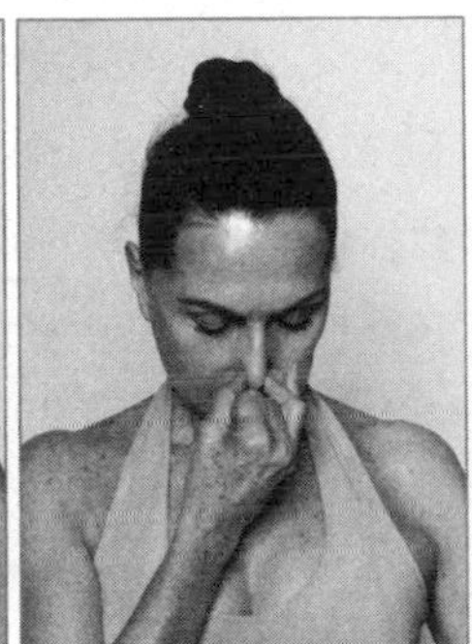
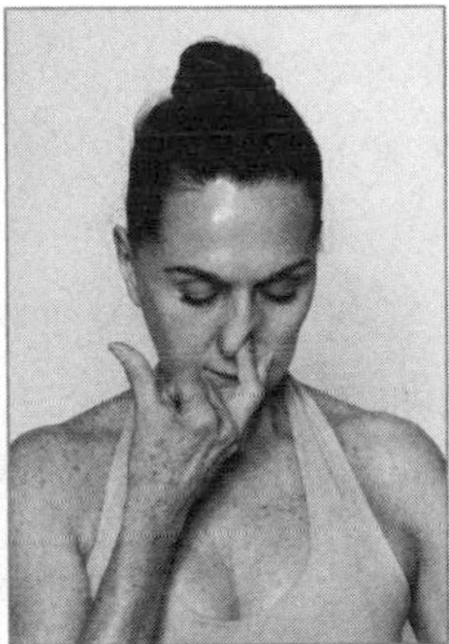
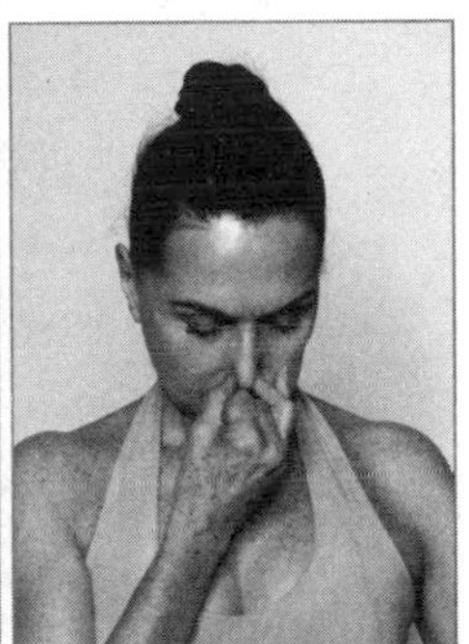

Be sure to hold mula bandha and jalandhara bandha throughout all four parts of the breath—while inhaling, while retaining the inhaled breath, while exhaling, and while retaining the exhaled breath (holding the breath out). Additionally, apply uddiyana bandha while retaining the exhaled breath. While the right hand is in vishnu mudra and is used to open and close the nostrils, use your left hand to keep track of the 7 rounds, counting on your fingers. And remember always to begin and end through the left nostril.

Option #1 (easier)*:* Instead of starting out by silently counting to 8, count to 2 instead, gradually increase to 4, then to 8.

Option #2 (more devotional)*:* Instead of silently counting with numbers, silently repeat a sacred Sanskrit mantra—for example, the 8-syllable mantra "*Shri Krishna Sharanam Mama*." Or choose an affirming phrase such as "May all be happy, may all be free" or "Let there be peace on earth."

Option #3 (more advanced)*:* Apply *kechari mudra* by curling the tongue back and pressing it up against the roof of the mouth and holding it there for the whole pranayama practice.

Option #4 (adding visualization): With each of the 7 rounds of the pranayama practice, visualize the seven main chakras—the doorways of perception—and their corresponding colors, moving from the root to the crown. Start with the first round, inhale into the left nostril, direct your prana to the site of the *muladhara* chakra at the base of the spine, and try to see a glowing, pulsating red orb. Continue to focus on the muladhara chakra throughout all of the four parts of the breath, making a full round, then focusing on the next chakra. Move, in order, from the root to the crown, focusing on each chakra and its corresponding color for a full round. Each time you start a round and enter into a chakra, feel that you are turning on a light switch in a dark room and actually see the color of the chakra pulsating.

1. Muladhara (base of spine): red
2. Swadhisthana (below the navel): orange
3. Manipura (at the solar plexus): yellow
4. Anahata (at the heart): green
5. Vishuddha (at the throat: blue
6. Anja (between the eyebrows): violet
7. Sahasrara (hovering over the top of the head): dazzling and clear like the color of diamonds

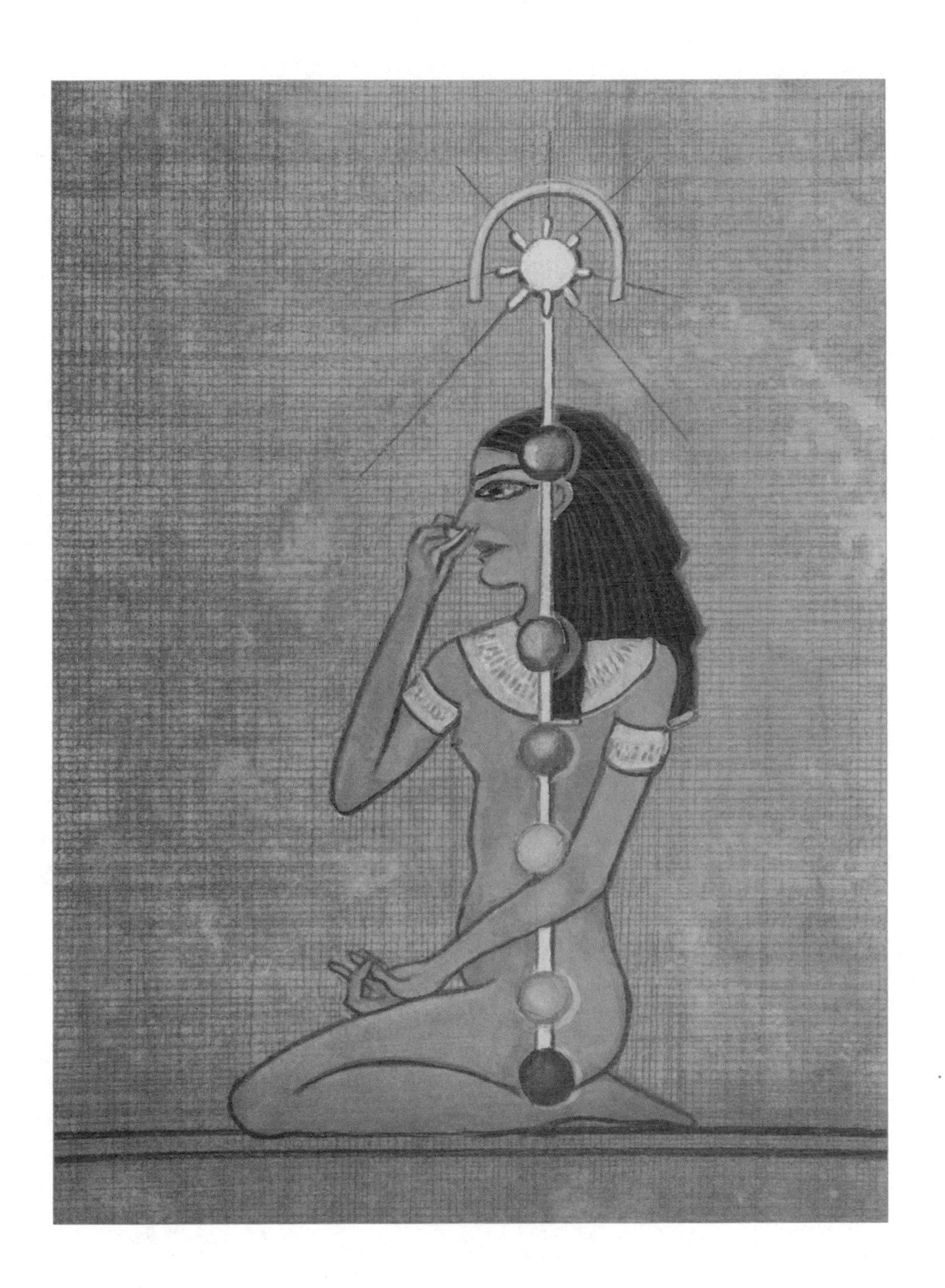

• WEEK 9 •

BEING THE WAY

MEDITATION

WEEK 9—Being the Way: Meditation

The hieroglyph of the bee designates both the bee and its honey, making it an appropriate symbol for meditation. Mastering the ability to concentrate takes effort, but the fruit of that effort arises gracefully as meditation, the state of sweet stillness.

My teacher Swami Nirmalananda often said, "Our main duty is to go beyond thought. Thoughts cause all sorts of problems. The true Self has no problems." Everyone wants to be free of problems and to feel confident and happy. True self-confidence comes from connecting to the unchanging eternal Self, the atman. Attachment to the movements of the mind results in a lack of self-confidence. False confidence is based in pride and arrogance, which are rooted in fear, not in the happiness of the soul. A changeable mind can never deliver calmness and stability or true happiness. A changeable mind is always grasping for the external material objects of the world. Patanjali, in his sutra *yogash chitta vritti nirodha PYS 1.2*, tells us that Yoga arises when we stop identifying with our thoughts, when we can let go of the fluctuations of our mind. To experience peace of mind we have to find a way to be free of thoughts, for at least a few moments, every day.

Meditation provides us with that freedom by connecting us to the eternal, unchanging reality within us. But don't expect to be able to empty your mind of thoughts. It is within the nature of the mind to think. The goal of meditation is not to "blank" your mind, the goal is to be able to let go of the mind's thoughts, to not be pulled into every thought that arises. Meditation develops the virtue of *sama*, which means "to calm," and therefore to be able to control the thoughts, the *chitta*—the whirlings of the mind. Sama enables one to be quiet, calm, and tranquil in the midst of the whirlings. By means of the steadiness of sama, when your mind gets distracted you can bring it back to a place of equanimity. A seasoned practitioner knows how to protect his or her innate serenity of mind—their *chitta prasadanam*, or blessed serene state of mind—through meditation.

When we are in deep sleep, we are free of thoughts. Scientists have observed this—there is no rapid eye movement (REM), so the conclusion is that the sleeper is not thinking, they have gone beyond thought, they are in deep sleep and are free of problems. The trick is to do this while you are awake—that's called meditation, or *dhyana* in Sanskrit.

Meditation is effortless and graceful, and you can't "make yourself" do it; it will arise on its own organically. But for that to happen, you have to apply effort and put in a lot of practice to develop your ability to focus your attention and not be easily distracted. For most of us, meditation practice is actually the practice of concentration. To be able to meditate you need to first develop *dharana*, the ability to concentrate, and for that you need to put in the hours; in other words, you must practice every day. Don't miss a day. Try to do it at the same time every day and, if possible, in the same place. Gradually over time you will get better at it. I promise you, if you stick with it, there will come a time when you will look forward to meditating and not think of it as something you should do because it is good for you.

Meditation practice is about moving toward the place where you reduce identification with your thoughts and experience a tranquil internal spacious reality. Meditation is the practice of focusing your mind—being able to let go of distractions and bring your attention back to your chosen object of focus. The mantra is a key component because it gives the restless mind something to do, or rather one thing to focus on, causing the barrage of thoughts to slow down, to begin to thin out.

There are many ways to meditate, hence the thousands of methods, types, or styles that have been handed down from many religious and spiritual traditions over the centuries. Generally speaking, all forms aim to let the practitioner watch his or her mind and let go of thinking. What differentiates the various methods is the object of focus. The object may be the breath, a visualization, a part of the body, a chakra, an inner light, or an external object like a candle or picture of a god, goddess, or saint. There are also forms of meditation where there is no one object to focus on; instead you keep the attention open as you witness your experience (as in Vipassana meditation). The best type of meditation is the one that works best for you, providing you with a way to calm your mind. The Jivamukti method of meditation is a mantra form of meditation, using the mantra "let go" as the focus.

This way to meditate, using the mantra "let go," developed for me quite organically. When I was eighteen years old and a high school student in Seattle, Washington, I attended a free talk about meditation. The lecturer presented a slide show to accompany his talk, showing various images of hectic human life in cities interspersed with natural scenes of placid lakes, sunsets, and vast open fields. He told us that the mind of a meditator was serene, calm, and peaceful and that this yogic state of mind was the natural state for a human being. He said that thoughts upset this natural state and that through meditation you could conquer these thoughts. His talk was very inspiring, but when I went home afterward I realized that he never actually taught us how to meditate, he only talked about the results of meditation. Still, I had a few things to go on—calmness and serenity were natural to the mind, thoughts were the enemy—so I decided to try it myself. I sat down in my room alone, closed my eyes, and tried to meditate. Of course, immediately one thought after the next bombarded me, grabbing my attention. Even "physical" thoughts started to make their demands—my nose started to inch, my lower back started to ache, and my right knee felt like it was going to explode. What to do? I started to talk to myself, saying the words "let go" over and over again. I stuck with it and the let-go mantra started to naturally align itself with my breath. As the inhale came, I said, "let," and with the exhale, "go." My attention became completely absorbed, so much so that over an hour went by during that first attempt. So every day I made it my project to practice letting go. At first I did it to prepare myself while I looked for a proper meditation teacher, but over the years it became the practice. Now over forty years later I am teaching it to others.

The power of meditation practice extends well beyond the actual time you sit every day. For example, the mantra "let go" can come in handy at other times. Try it when you find yourself in a challenging situation at work or at home when someone is trying your patience. When you find that your mind is becoming disturbed and losing its calmness and you are on the verge of reacting to the agitation with an angry, spiteful comment, remember the mantra and silently say, "Let go." Immediately you will feel the positive effect—you remain calm, neutral, and cool, better able to handle the situation. When experiences like this happen, you are taking the benefits of your meditation off the cushion and into the world.

There isn't a lot you need to have to practice meditation besides a method and a place to sit. How you sit for meditation is important because you don't want discomforts of the body to distract your focus. To be able to calm your mind and go beyond thoughts it is helpful to find a good, comfortable way to sit that works for you. We have all seen the classical images of yogis sitting in a lotus posture, and ancient scriptures like the *Hatha Yoga Pradipika* do suggest that the best posture for meditation is padmasana. But what if you can't cross your legs like that? Can you still practice meditation? Yes. There are various seated postures; even sitting on a chair is an acceptable way to meditate. Please refer to Week 8, Directing the Way: Pranayama, for detailed explanations of several seated positions that can be used for meditation. Also, you may want to reference my book with David Life, *Jivamukti Yoga: Practices for Liberating Body and Soul*, chapter 10, in which you will find pictures of several seated asanas that can be good for meditation practice.

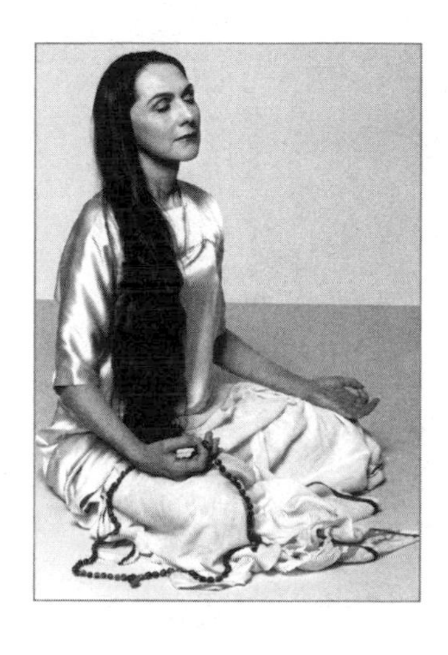

THE PRACTICE

THREE STEPS: 1. CHOOSE YOUR SEAT.
2. BE STILL. 3. FOCUS.

1. **Choose your seat.** Select a comfortable seated position. You may even wish to sit against the wall or in a chair. It is important that the spine be perpendicular to the Earth. If you are sitting on the floor, elevate the seat by sitting on a pillow or folded blanket. You must be able to sit still for the duration of the practice, so don't choose a position that is too challenging.

   Begin by placing your feet, legs, and hips in the most comfortable position available. Relax. Sit easily. Feel your seat as it connects to the floor—sit down. Surrender to the terrestrial force by feeling the force of gravity drawing your seat downward. As you surrender to this downward force you will automatically feel an uplifting force moving through your spine and torso. This is the force of levitation operating within you. As you sit down you will be lifted up. Relax your hands and place them comfortably on your knees, palms up or down or in your lap. If your hands are in your lap, place your active hand on top of your other hand, with both palms up. Relax your arms and shoulders. Feel your neck soften and lengthen. Relax your face. Gently close your eyes. Allow your chin to be level with the floor as you release your jaw. Let your tongue float inside your mouth. Relax lips, cheeks, nose, eyes, inside your nose and behind your eyes, eyebrows, and forehead. Allow the frontal part of your brain to slip back slightly into the skull. Relax your scalp. Scan the body over and make any adjustments you feel you need to make so that you have the most comfortable seat and then . . .

2. **Be still.** Once you have chosen your seat, do not doubt your choice. Don't move the body; let go of any urge to fidget or adjust your position; just stay as you are. Our normal reaction to anything uncomfortable is to move away from it. By allowing the body to be still you override your normal reactionary, habitual ways of dealing with discomfort. The benefit here is that you develop the ability to take a fragmented mind that is distracted by every little thing and pull your attention to a concentrated focus.
3. **Focus.** Mantra provides the focus. Silently repeat the mantra "let go" with the passing of each breath. Breathe in "let," breathe out "go." Don't try to breathe in any special way; in fact don't actively breathe. Instead, allow the breath to "breathe your body" while you watch from the place of the nonjudgmental witness, the *sakshi*. Become the witness of breathing. Let the breath come and let it go. In a short time your thoughts will begin to align themselves with the flow of the breath. The breath comes into the body as a thought comes into the mind. Let that thought pass through your mind as you let the breath pass through the body. Let there to be a continuous movement of breath through the body and thoughts through the mind while you let go of identification with your body and mind by letting go of each breath and each thought.

Note of encouragement: During the practice you may lose your concentration, become distracted, and wander off with a thought. This is normal for a meditator. When you become aware that this has occurred, gently bring your attention back to the mantra and continue to concentrate on letting each breath and each thought come and go. With each letting go, the mind begins to recede back into its source, the same source that our consciousness retreats to during deep sleep. But unlike the sleeper, the meditator is awake and conscious of this process. He or she is witnessing it. By identifying with the sakshi, the witness, you let go of all that is impermanent—that which has within its nature to move and change. What will remain is the unchanging eternal Self: the indwelling atman, beyond the body and mind. By letting go, you let God.

Be patient. Don't expect results overnight. Meditation demands continuous practice over a long period of time. But if you sincerely commit to the practice, the results will emerge organically and gracefully.

HOW LONG SHOULD YOU PRACTICE?

Option #1 (easier)*:* Use a timer. In the beginning, when you are first establishing a meditation practice, set the timer for 5 minutes. Try to master 5 minutes. Then increase by small increments. For example, every week, increase your practice by 1 minute until you can sit comfortably and meditate silently repeating the mantra "let go" for 20–30 minutes.

Option #2 (more traditional)*:* Use a mala (prayer beads, rosary) to keep track of the time spent in meditation. Decide beforehand how many rounds you are going to do and then stick to that number. For example, decide you will meditate for the time it takes you to go around one mala, holding each bead between the thumb and ring finger of the right hand, while silently repeating the mantra "let go." Always use your right hand to move the beads, resting your left hand comfortably either in your lap or on your left thigh.

Option #3 (more devotional)*:* Mentally recite a mantra that contains the name of God. The more mystical mantras, which have the name of God embedded in their formula, work like magical spells to transport you out of the mundane world into a *leela* realm—a parallel divine dimension where bliss reigns supreme. The name of God is the same as God. So by saying God's name you invoke the presence of God.

Mantras are not loaded with conventional meaning; they vibrate with *essential* meaning. Sanskrit mantras in particular are believed to be sound expressions of the consciousness of the Divine—the subtle forms of God, so that when you recite them you have an opportunity to link with God. Through mantra you have the means to identify with a specific deity or with reality itself. But the mere repetition of a mantra will not necessarily have a spiritualizing effect. Traditionally a qualified teacher, someone who had personally experienced the power of the mantra, gives a mantra to a student, thereby making the mantra more potent. But there is no harm, and potentially much to gain, by reciting a mantra before you feel ready to ask for initiation from a teacher.

Some Sanskrit mantras you might want to practice with are: the 3-syllable mantra *Hari Om*, inhaling *Hari*, exhaling *Om*; the 6-syllable mantra *Om Namah Shivaya*, inhaling *Om Namah* and exhaling *Shivaya*; the 8-syllable mantra *Shri Krishna Sharanam Mama*, inhaling *Shri Krishna*, exhaling *Sharanam Mama*: the 16-syllable mantra *Hare Krishna Hare Krishna / Krishna Krishna Hare Hare / Hare Rama Hare Rama / Rama Rama Hare Hare*, inhaling *Hare Krishna Hare Krishna*, exhaling *Krishna Krishna Hare Hare*, inhaling *Hare Rama Hare Rama*, exhaling *Rama Rama Hare Hare*. The mantra doesn't necessarily have to be divided between inhale and exhale. You could repeat the entire mantra on the inhale and then again on the exhale, or you could let go of attempting to coordinate your breath with the mantra and instead allow the mantra to penetrate internally as you quiet yourself and listen for the mantra to sound itself.

Traditionally yogis used a mala as a meditation tool, to keep track of counting while reciting a mantra. Holding each bead and silently reciting a mantra is called *japa* meditation. *Japa* means "mantra repetition"; you continue to recite the same mantra over and over, using the mala to maintain your focus. When you get to the end of the mala, there may be a tail or a tassel and a larger bead, traditionally called the "guru" bead. You should never pass over the guru bead; instead flip the mala around and start over from the other end. Malas are usually strung with 108 beads (excluding the guru bead) or some division of that number, for example 54, 27, or 18. You should do as many rounds as you feel you have time for.

• WEEK 10 •

GIVING AWAY

RELAXATION

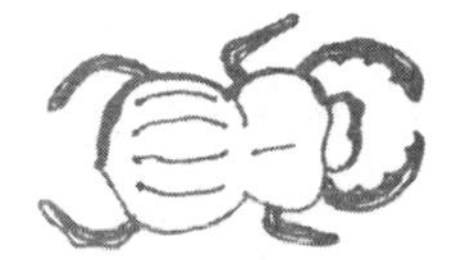

WEEK 10—Giving Away: Relaxation

There was great interest in life after death in ancient Egypt. The scarab is associated with death and resurrection and symbolizes the movement of the sun across the sky, representing the soul's journey through life and death. If we observe how the Egyptians positioned their dead, we see that it is similar to shavasana, rather than in a fetal position or lying on one side or on the abdomen or seated, and often with a scarab protecting the heart.

The secret to success in yoga is to give away the benefits you have achieved through your hard work—not to hold on to them for yourself. *Shavasana* means "the seat of the corpse." It is a yoga practice of deep relaxation, actually designed to prepare you for death, for letting go of your body. If you practice it daily, you will undoubtedly be better prepared for death, but also you will be able to live more relaxed and at ease with your life, because the practice, by helping you overcome the fear of death, provides the key to living a grace-filled life.

Patanjali speaks of *abhinivesha*—the fear of death—as one of the five *kleshas*, or obstacles to Yoga. The fear of death, as well as all other fears, comes down to the fear of losing. Unless we have some spiritual training, it is very difficult to overcome the fear of death—of losing our life, of losing our body. Regular practice of deep relaxation diminishes our identification with the body, resulting in fearlessness.

To relax means to become receptive. When you relax, you let go of trying to control everything. You stop doing, stop talking, planning, judging, figuring things out, and instead listen and receive. You surrender your body, mind, intelligence, and sense of self to a higher power, a higher Self. But there is no need to surrender as in defeat; true yogic surrender is to devote yourself to the Divine Eternal Source—that which is infinite love. To relax is to let go and let God.

The body is very receptive to suggestion. In fact, the power of your own mental suggestion is the most powerful force working upon you. By suggesting relaxation, you concentrate your mental powers in a positive way toward your physical body. Great healing can take place on many levels through this practice of deep relaxation. Physical illness can be banished from the body, as can mental disease. It is a rejuvenating, healing practice, which results in a more positive outlook, more enthusiasm for life, and a willingness to make the best of every moment. Relaxation is definitely the yogi's way.

THE PRACTICE

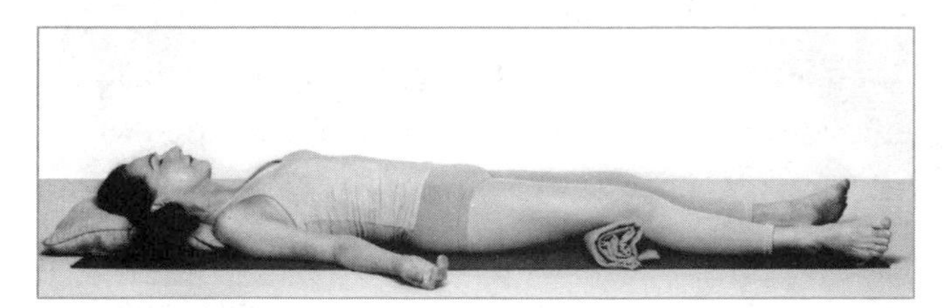

Prepare by lying down on your back. Place a pillow under your head to allow your jaw and neck to release and a rolled-up blanket or bolster under your knees to allow your lower back to release. Before moving deeper into relaxation it is helpful to consciously create tension in the body. Do this by making fists with your hands and clenching your feet, lifting your legs, arms, and head off the floor, and scrunching your facial muscles into a "prune face." Hold everything in tension for a few seconds, then release back to the floor. Stick out your tongue and exhale, relax your mouth, allowing the jaw to go slack. Open your legs wider than hip width and allow your feet to turn out. Place your arms along the sides of your body, palms up, with your shoulder blades releasing to the floor. Close your eyes gently and let your breath come passively.

Consciously suggest relaxation to every body part, starting with your toes and slowly moving upward while silently saying, "Toes relax, feet relax, legs relax, hips relax, lower back relax, middle back relax, upper back relax, abdomen relax, chest relax, fingers relax, hands relax, arms relax, shoulders relax, neck and throat relax, face relax, lips and mouth relax, tongue relax, cheeks relax, nose relax, eyes relax, forehead relax, head and scalp relax, organs of elimination relax, organs of sexuality relax, organs of digestion relax, organs of circulation relax, organs of respiration relax, organs of sense and feeling relax, organs of thinking relax. My whole body, inside and out, is completely relaxed."

> *Option* (more devotional): Concentrate on giving your all to God. Start with your toes and silently say (as if you were talking to God, using your own personal name for the divine, e.g., Goddess, Christ, Allah, Jehovah, Krishna, etc.), "These toes, I give them to you, my Lord Krishna. These feet, take them, they are yours, and these ankles are yours, take them. These legs and hips are yours, this back is yours, this abdomen and chest is yours, these fingers and hands are yours, and these arms and shoulders are yours. This neck and throat is yours. This face is your face, dear Lord, take it. This head is yours, take it. All of my internal organs are yours, the organs of elimination are yours, the organs of sexuality are yours, my stomach and other organs of digestion are yours, my heart is yours, my lungs are yours, my skin is yours, dear Lord. All of my senses are yours, my sense of smell, taste, sight, touch, and hearing are yours, my emotions, mind, intelligence, consciousness, and my sense of self is yours. My very soul is yours, dear Lord, take me, I am yours."

A STORY

ORIGINALLY, THIS BOOK WAS INTENDED to be a technical manual detailing the spiritual practices that I do at home in the morning. After I had written the first draft, I showed it to my partner, David Life, and asked his opinion. He read it and said that while it was clear and detailed in such a way that most people would be able to follow it and derive benefit from it, he felt that it was a bit dry.

"Dry—what do you mean by dry?" I asked.

"Well, it lacks mystery and magic—the very things that make yoga attractive to people," David wisely said.

"What do you suggest, then, to give it more of a mystique?"

"You need a story to share with your readers about how you came up with *The Magic Ten and Beyond*."

"But that was so long ago, and so personal, and there are so many holes in the story—and most people won't believe it," I protested.

"Yes, but all of that is the reason you should tell the story."

"Really?"

"Yes."

"Does it have to be completely factual?"

"Facts don't always make for a good story."

"Okay, then . . ."

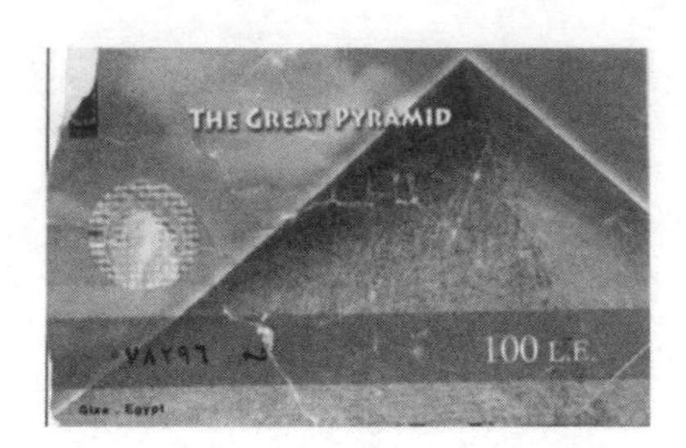

Admission ticket stub for the Great Pyramid

Here's the story . . .

"What are you doing, Sharon?" David says. "Shh!" I whisper, beckoning David to come closer and cover me as I place my right hand and left foot on the broken lower edge of the cold stone sarcophagus. David stares skeptically and shakes his head no as I climb, then slip silently into the granite coffer and lie down on my back. Feeling confined by the sides of the box, I automatically fold my arms pharaonic-style over my chest, close my eyes, still my body, and relax.

We are in Egypt, in the King's Chamber of the Great Pyramid at Giza. There are only a couple of other tourists with us, and, surprisingly, no museum guards. So with David as my lookout, I'm determined to make the most of this rare privilege, not knowing how much time I have.

First there is the sound experience.

The humming, which seems to be coming from inside the stone itself, sounds like billions of bees industriously focused on some altruistic work. Across my eyelids flash images of Napoleon's golden bees—interestingly, the symbol he chose for his empire after he returned to Paris from his expedition to Egypt, where, by his own accounts, he had a mystical experience while spending the night in the King's Chamber of the Great Pyramid. Is there a connection? I wonder if he heard the bees, too. I consciously stop myself from going off on a Napoleonic tangent and return to the project of relaxing. As the images soften, I descend into a meditative place of deep listening. The humming becomes intense; my body seems to be floating in the box. I sense a space between my skin and the smoothness of the stone, and I realize that my body is not touching stone—it is touching sound. The molecules of my body

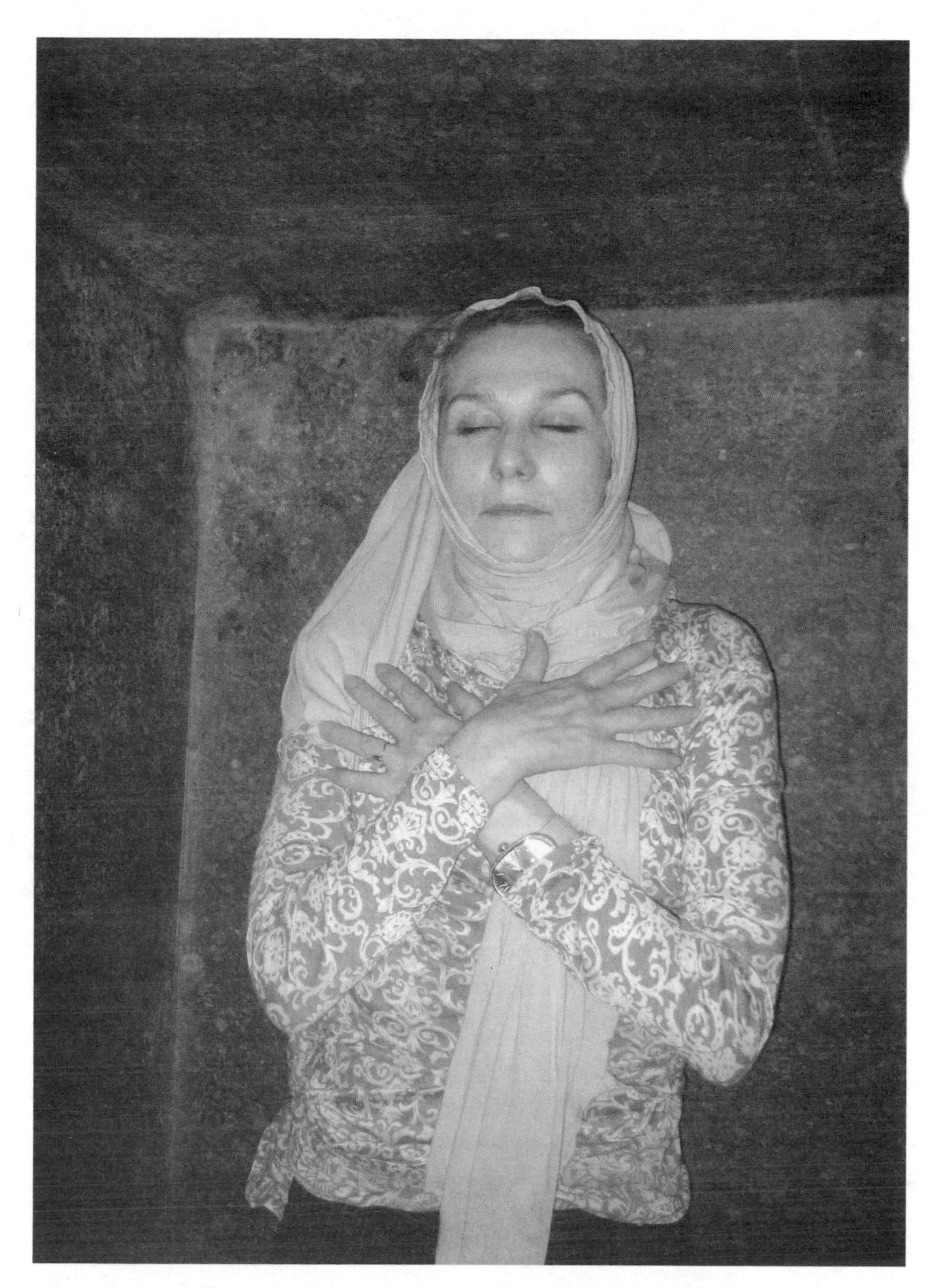

The author lying in the sarcophagus in the King's Chamber

are resonating with the molecules of the stone and the space in between. I feel comfortable and at ease. I get that familiar feeling of déjà vu and know that I have been here before. "Just let go a bit more," I tell myself as I exhale. And then there is a surge of energy from my solar plexus, accompanied by the sensation of taking off. I feel as if my soul has wings and is lifting up, flying out of my body.

Suddenly my perspective changes and I feel myself suspended near the ceiling of the chamber. I look down and see someone lying in the coffer. I know that she has been there for some days, maybe a week, in a state close to hibernation; the beating of the heart has slowed, and with it the breath. Someone who didn't know might think this person was dead, but I know that she is not dead. She is in retreat—undergoing some type of initiation. She is a student of an esoteric mystery school, lying in a meditative trance brought about through intense yogic practices over a long period of time. As I gaze at her, the middle of her torso begins to rise up, until only her hands and feet are touching the bottom of the coffer. Could she have been me, in another life?

Just then a flash of light closes the window to another time. A tourist has hovered over me and taken a picture of me in the sarcophagus. Then David helps me out and we sit on the stone floor of the King's Chamber as I tell him about my out-of-body experience—the bees and the vision. Then, even though I am a bit shaken, we make our way out of the King's Chamber by going back the way we came in, through what is known as the "thieves' entrance"—a rough hole in the side of the pyramid made with a battering ram in AD 820. We hold on to the rope banisters that line the ramp—planks of wood that form the walkway into and out of the pyramid. At times we have to all but crawl through dark, narrow passages that seem to ethereally glow and pulsate. Eventually we do make it out into the bright sun and heat of the desert, feeling like we have been reborn.

The next day we are wandering amid sarcophagi, mummies, immense stone sculptures, cobwebs, layers of dust, and sleepy guards in the exhibition rooms of the Egyptian Museum in Cairo. I spot a section of an ancient temple wall painted with brightly colored figures and hieroglyphs. I walk closer to inspect an upside-down female figure who appears to be performing a yoga asana known in Sanskrit as *urdhva dhanurasana*—often referred to as wheel pose in English.

"Wow! She's doing yoga!"

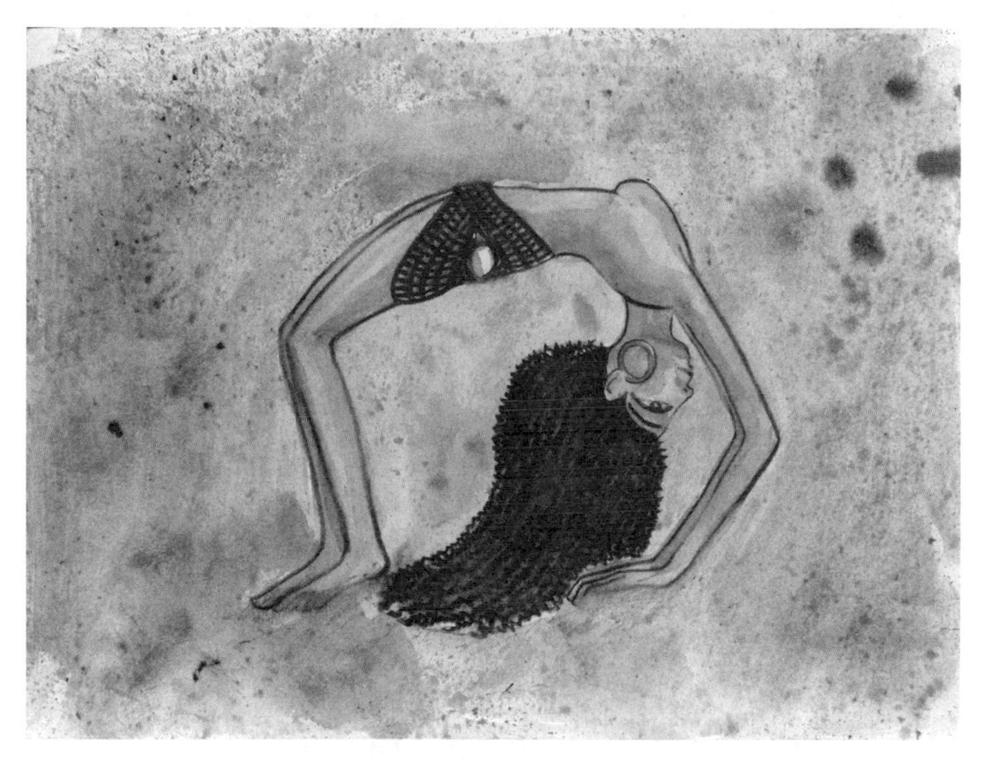

Egyptian yogini in wheel

I excitedly look for David, who I find in the next room, bending over a glass case filled with a collection of gold toe and finger casings. Both of us are incredulous, not so much because of the priceless objects but because of how flimsy the case is. It's a rectangular box made of thin pieces of glass, framed with fragile pieces of wood. There's a small latch, which is held closed by a piece of twisted wire. On top of the glass is a small strip of yellowed notebook paper with an even more yellowed piece of Scotch tape attaching the paper to the glass. Typed on the paper are the following words identifying the contents:

GOLD PROTECTORS FOUND ON THE FINGERS AND TOES OF THE MUMMY OF KING TUTANKHAMEN.

As we look up from the display we notice that the room is filled with many glass cases like this one, housing priceless, irreplaceable objects, and that all the windows in the room are open, letting in dust, heat, and pollution from the street outside. We both think: "Where are the humidifiers, the security system, the guards? If these things were in the Metropolitan Museum of Art they would definitely be protected better, like gold in Fort Knox, rather than like costume jewelry."

"David, I want to show you something really interesting," I say, and I lead him back to the room where the "yoga" painting is. We are standing there looking at it and I say, "Do you think it's possible that the roots of yoga could be found in ancient Egypt and not be the sole property of India, or at any rate had been available to both ancient cultures at the same time?"

"Sure, why not?" he says. "We too often take as fact what a few historians have said, but no one really knows the truth about the past—for the most part it is all speculation. But besides this painting of someone doing the wheel, do you have any other evidence that might support your theory?"

I have to admit that I only have an intuitive feeling—no provable facts. But still the idea holds me; the possible connection between yoga and Egypt has captivated me since I was young and became attracted to all things magical and mystical. Although I have never come across anyone who believed that yoga was practiced in ancient Egypt, or even considered the possibility, while reading about ancient Egypt I have often come across references to "ancient Egyptian mystery schools." What might have been taught in those schools indeed remains a mystery, although many people have speculated on the possibilities. The Western hermetic tradition claims to have descended from the Egyptian mystery schools and cites the Egyptian god Thoth, also known as Hermes Trismegistus, as the source of the occult knowledge embraced by many modern secret societies, such as the Rosicrucian Fellowship and the Theosophists. Many great thinkers, scientists, and alchemists, including Pythagoras, Paracelsus, Sir Isaac Newton, and Ralph Waldo Emerson, acknowledged the occult wisdom of ancient Egypt.

Legend says that it was very difficult to be accepted into the ancient mystery schools. A prospective student would have to pass arduous initiation tests in places like the King's Chamber of the Great Pyramid to prove he or she was qualified. Then what? What were students taught to practice in these schools after gaining entry? Once again, we have no concrete evidence—no old textbooks have yet to be unearthed at archaeological digs—but we do know that the ancients burned with the same quest to know the truth as we do today. To know who we really are, and what our purpose is here on Earth—these are universal questions shared by all spiritual traditions.

The Bible talks about Egyptian priests as wise men who were able to perform magic, make themselves invisible, and cast spells by uttering incantations or mantras. Many ancient yogic scriptures describe similar accomplishments as a result of yoga practices. The Indian scriptures provide the scholar with a wealth of knowledge, but to the adventurous practitioner they provide applicable methods, "technologies of ecstasy" in the phrase used by the scholar Alain Daniélou, to describe the transcendental experiential practices of yoga that go beyond intellectual speculation. But the point is, India wrote down its systems of yoga, and those writings still exist today, whereas no clearly written evidence of a yoga system has been unearthed in Egypt—at least not yet.

We do know that the Egyptians invented paper and were very committed to writing and to the refinement of written language, which we see in the pictorial language of hieroglyphs. There were actually scribe schools, vocational schools devoted to teaching students how to write. Scribes were sought after and employed in many different areas of Egyptian society. It is highly probable that texts were written describing practices that were taught in the mystery schools, practices that would enable someone to do what might appear to ordinary people to be magic—or yoga. Many of those texts might have been stored in the great Library of Alexandria.

"You've always had the intuition that the ancient Egyptians had schools where they practiced meditation and yoga-type techniques," David continues. "They were obviously very interested in preservation and were prolific writers and maintained large libraries. There may have been instructional texts describing the practices. But I guess we will never know for sure because weren't all the libraries destroyed? I definitely remember from high school history class that Julius Caesar burned a large library at Alexandria."

"Yes, you're right," a voice says.

We turn to face an elegantly dressed middle-aged man with a shaved head and piercing blue eyes that convey lots of mischief. He says, "But the library was actually burned several times before Caesar and not always by Romans, so we can't blame the Romans for destroying everything!"

He bows low and, slowly coming to an upright posture, introduces himself. "My name is Karim Hassan. I'm an Egyptologist and work here at the museum. Pardon me, but I overheard your conversation about yoga, magic, and Egypt. Are you yoga practitioners?"

"Yes," we say, and introduce ourselves.

"I don't meet very many yogis here in Cairo. Are you from America—I think your accent is American?"

"Yes, New York City."

"Hmm, New York City. Very good. You have tall buildings. What do you do there?"

"We teach yoga."

"Ahh . . . interesting. Are you just visiting Cairo as tourists?"

"Yes, basically, but we do have an interest in ancient Egypt from a spiritual perspective."

"How do you mean?"

"Mr. Hassan . . . ," I begin.

"Please, call me Karim."

"Karim, do you think that yoga could have been practiced in ancient Egypt? Do you think the yoga practices might have been taught in the mystery schools?"

Karim laughs. "This is a very interesting hypothesis," he says. "Tell me, what do you know of these mystery schools?"

"We don't know anything, really," David says. "Sharon has always had a feeling, that's all. Do you know anything about these mystery schools—did they even exist?"

"How long are you in Cairo?"

"Just a few more days."

"Hmm . . . that's too bad, as I am enjoying your company; but okay, we can make this work, and as they say in our country, 'As long as the sun is in the sky, it's daytime!' May I show you something that I think may be of interest to you?"

"Yes, of course. We are honored that you are even thinking about our interests," I reply.

“Splendid, but you must come with me to my office. I will warn you, though, it is underneath the museum and very much like a tomb. I hope you aren’t claustrophobic.”

We follow Karim through the museum’s galleries and down some dimly lit stairs into the basement, where his office is. Karim opens the door and switches on a light. It is a windowless room, very elegantly and comfortably arranged, resembling an apartment more than an office.

“Please, may I offer you some tea? I’ve just returned from Paris, where I was introduced to a wonderful oolong tea while visiting a lovely teashop in the Louvre.”

“Yes, we would love some tea.”

He motions to us to sit on the floor, where plush cushions are arranged around a low Moroccan-style carved table. The stone floor is covered with a soft Oriental carpet. The room smells clean and is cool, calm, and extremely quiet—a marked difference from the busy museum upstairs and certainly an oasis from the chaos outside on the streets.

“It’s cool and quiet down here—the walls are thick, 304 centimeters—that’s about ten feet of stone,” Karim explains. “I’ve worked for the museum a long time, so seniority does provide a few perks. I spend a lot of hours here, so it is nice that the office is comfortable.”

Karim holds a tin of tea in each hand and, nodding to his right, says, “This oolong tea is blended with pea flowers and when brewed turns a heavenly sky-blue color—quite exceptional, really.” Then, nodding to his left, he says, “Or would you prefer some nice Egyptian peppermint—more traditional?” But without giving us a chance to speak, he puts the peppermint tea down and decides with a smile, “Let’s try the blue, shall we?”

He fills an electric teakettle with bottled water and, as he begins to organize our tea party, asks us, “Please tell me more about your ideas.”

“Well,” I begin, “the gist of it is, I’ve felt that perhaps we have been too ready to accept India as the birthplace of yoga, when maybe yoga is more universal and might have appeared in other ancient cultures as well. Perhaps yoga was practiced in Egypt at the same time or even predating India. Please don’t get me wrong—I love India. Still, I can’t deny that I am attracted to the mysteries of ancient Egypt. Perhaps I want to reconcile this by finding some evidence that yoga might have been shared by both cultures. India gets the credit for yoga, and rightly so. The Indians refined, codified, and documented the methods, making them accessible to anyone who had an interest and could decipher the language and immerse himself or herself in the practices. The philosophy and methods have been kept alive for thousands of years, passed down from guru to disciple.

"The Egyptians, on the other hand, seem to have been very good at burying their spiritual secrets, whether deliberately or inadvertently. The spiritual writings of India have survived the centuries, whereas much of the Egyptian wisdom seems to have been lost, stolen, destroyed, or embedded in a language of hieroglyphics that has yet to be fully cracked."

"Do you feel that a form of yoga was taught in the mystery schools of ancient Egypt?" Karim asks while looking directly at me, and I flash back to my out-of-body experience in the King's Chamber the day before.

"Do you believe in karma and reincarnation?" Karim asks.

"Yes."

"Do you know about your past lives?"

"No."

"But you do feel that you have lived before, a long time ago, in Egypt, and that you were an initiate in one of these mystery schools?" Karim suggests.

The pot begins to whistle. "Ah, here's our tea!" Karim says.

As he attends to the tea, David and I, in awe of the incredible luck that led to meeting this fascinating man, look at each other, our eyes wide, as if to say, "What have we stumbled upon here?"

After letting the tea steep, Karim places the tea tray on the low table and, while pouring us each a steaming, fragrant cup, continues: "Did you know that Egypt was not always the name of our country? The ancient Greeks called our land Khem, which means 'black,' as in rich, fertile soil in which anything can grow. They used to say that our ancient people lived in such a fertile environment that all they had to do was envision what they wanted and it would magically appear. *Khem* is the root of the word 'chemistry,' which is defined as the ability to work with the elements. The Arabic prefix *al* was added to *khem* to make the word 'alchemy,' the magical art of transformation. Ancient Egypt was the land of magical transformation. There *were* esoteric schools that taught these magical arts. These magical arts deal with the knowledge of how things work, how every action plants a seed and seeds sprout and grow into reality. It is wise to know the laws of karma, because then you can participate, you know—consciously direct your destiny—that sort of thing." He smiles and suggests, "Let's sit for a moment and drink in the delicate flavors of this most exquisite blue tea."

A few minutes pass and then Karim speaks again. "Even though your speculations are interesting, I am not sure there exists enough evidence to prove that yoga, as you think of it—the poses, and so forth—originated in Egypt. But as a scholar I have discovered some intriguing things. For example, in the museum upstairs, the painting of the girl bending backward that attracted your attention today . . . did you know that our Egyptian numbering is decimal, broken up into units of tens? The tens are reckoned with a symbol that looks like an upside-down U from the English alphabet and the letter Ω, omega, in the Greek."

Karim lifts his eyebrows and pauses to make sure we are following him and then continues.

"I ask you now to envision the painting and consider this: our pictorial hieroglyphs reveal a language of symbols. The inverted bow shape of the upside-down girl is the same shape as the glyph for our number ten. Most of our hieroglyphs have more than one meaning—in this case, the same symbol for ten is also used to mean a harness, which oxen or bulls would wear when pulling carts or plowing fields—a yoke. Can you see how it could look like that?"

"What? 'Yoga' means 'to yoke'!" I can't contain my excitement. "This is way too much of a coincidence. The upside-down U means a ten as well as a yoke, wow!"

Karim says, "Well, anyway, the number ten does seem to have been a magical number for our ancients."

"Karim, we are intrigued—but magic? What do you mean by magic and magical numbers?"

"Well, let me ask you, what is your understanding of magic? Conjuring tricks? Pulling rabbits out of hats, sawing people in half? That kind of thing? Our ancients saw the world as a magical manifestation. We approached magic as a practical art to be used as a kind of applied science. The holders of this knowledge were shape-shifters who knew how to apply this wisdom to all areas of life, including farming, medicine, music, mathematics, astronomy, and architecture. But at the core was always the highest application—to transform the person into his or her ultimate potential."

"Which is what?" David asks.

"Immortality, of course," Karim states decisively. "You must have heard about our great radical religious reformer, Pharaoh Akhenaten."

"Yes, of course—he was the husband of Nefertiti and the father of the famous boy-king Tutankhamen," I offer.

"Do you know anything else?" he asks me patiently.

"Yes. I have actually done a bit of research. He was *satyagraha*—'possessed by the truth'—even more so than Gandhi. He believed that God, truth, and the sun were one and lived inside of him as his immortal soul."

"There is a phrase that occurs over and over, a kind of slogan credited to Akhenaten," Karim says, "that sums up his political aim: 'Living in *maet*.' *Maet* means truth—as in Divine Truth. Akhenaten saw God as the sun radiating light, compassionately illuminating all of us on Earth and more so, that we were meant to be vessels for this light. He directed his artists to create paintings and sculptures in which the sun is shown as a person with arms made of rays tapering into exquisite humanlike hands, extending downward to Earth, shining on the royal family, who exemplified living in the light."

"He saw himself as the son of the sun," I say, "and he went so far as to look upon the wearing of clothes as deceitful—he saw it as hiding from the truth, or from the sun. He himself became a nudist and required his family to go naked so as to be more truthful. He, his wife, and their daughters would appear publicly without clothes as an example to the people. He even felt that to live in houses was not truthful—as if doing so was hiding from the sun."

"His ideas seemed to be aligned with the homeless sky-clad, or naked, yogis mentioned in Vedic literature. His ideas were very radical and unpopular, and he may have been assassinated for them," David adds.

"Yes, it is true—unfortunately he was way ahead of his time," Karim says. "Do you know that he created a new religion, with the sun being the one God? And you could say that he created his own logo by altering the way the word for sun was written.

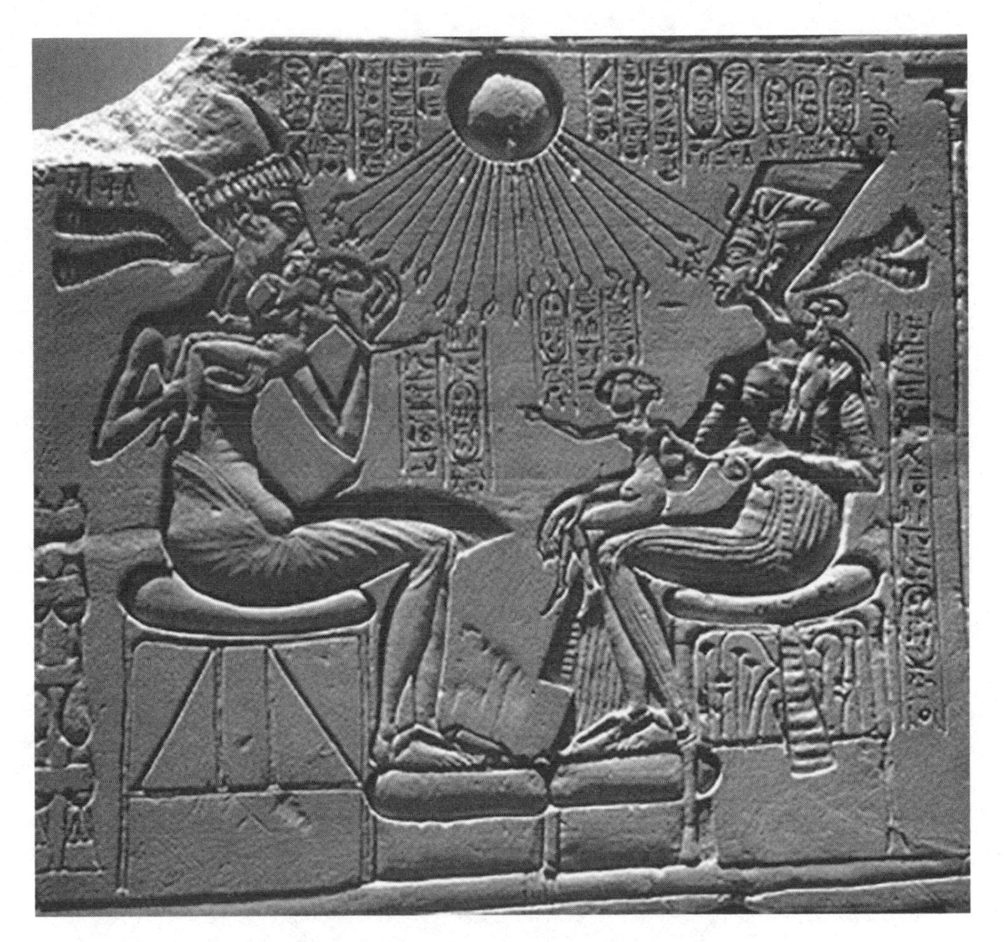

The sun radiating light upon the pharaoh and his family

Before him the hieroglyph for the sun was a simple disc. He added a dot in the center of that circle. That dot was symbolic of the soul."

Barely restraining my excitement, I say, "Yes, the eternal soul—like the Indian atman, the Self within the self."

"There's more. He changed his name from Amenhotep IV to Akhenaten. His new name was highly charged with meaning. It translates as 'the place where God rests or resides.' *Akh* means 'to live' and *aten*, 'the sun.' He saw himself, his body, as providing the place for God to live. He is saying with his name that he embodies truth, the light, the sun."

"*Aten* means 'the sun' and it also means the one God? I think this means he was enlightened, that he realized the atman—the Divine Self within himself. So could you say that he called himself Akhenaten to express that he was living liberated? This is exciting, because it sounds very close to the yogic concept of the *jivanmukta*—'one who lives liberated.'"

Karim nods appreciatively and we sit in silence for a few minutes. Then he says, "I'd like to show you something that the museum has recently acquired. I've been given the job of authenticating it, and, well, let me show you . . ."

Karim stands up slowly, and with a gentle downward motion of his hands indicates that we should remain seated. "Slowly sip, don't rush. When will you get an opportunity again to savor a moment such as this? You're in exotic Cairo—a place of ancient magic and mystery. We Egyptians move at a slower pace than you Americans. Perhaps it's the heat, or maybe just the dryness, and we are reluctant to stir up dust. It is a fact that we live in the shade of massive unmovable stone pyramids; we like things settled, and we don't like to unsettle things." Karim walks toward a large antique wooden desk in front of a wall of floor-to-ceiling books. He sits down on the chair behind the desk, which faces into the room. He pulls open a drawer and extracts a small metal box. "Ah, yes, here's the key," he says. "Would you be so kind as to excuse me for a moment?"

Karim opens a door into a room to the right of his desk and closes it behind him, leaving us sitting alone in his quiet office. After a minute or so I joke, "Do you think he has a mummy in there?"

"Maybe ten of them!" David smiles.

After a few minutes Karim reappears, places a folder on his desk, and invites us to come over and have a look. He apologizes and says that he can't show us the original, for security reasons, and that what we are looking at is a photograph of a cartouche. His job is to authenticate it, which means both to date it and to decipher its meaning.

"What you are looking at is a cartouche—carved in relief on the top of a box that was found at an archaeological dig in the tomb of an as yet unidentified mummy in the remains of Amarna, the city that Akhenaten built, so that makes it at least three thousand years old. You've seen cartouches before? A cartouche is a ring that magically protects what is inside it. It's a magic circle, but the circular form has been elongated and transformed into an oval, so that the hieroglyphs can be more easily contained. The hieroglyphic writing is encircled with something that looks like a rope and is tied at the end. The circle and tie are magical elements always found in a cartouche."

"Please explain what this cartouche means," I ask. "What is the magic in it—can you translate the hieroglyphs for us?"

"A cartouche usually identifies a person, often a pharaoh, but this one is communicating more than just a name. It could be a protection prayer or a magical formula. So far, from what I can tell, this one seems to be more of a formula. Here, let me show you. At the top there is the glyph for the number ten, which as we have mentioned can also mean 'yoke.'"

"Or maybe 'yoga'?" I offer.

Karim shrugs and continues: "Underneath it is the disc with a dot in the center, Akhenaten's symbol for the aten. Then, as we can see, there are ten symbols arranged in two columns. Starting from the top left and moving down, we have the radiating sun, two uplifted arms representing spirit or the *ka,* or 'soul,' an outstretched arm with an offering in the hand, a chair, and a dancer. Then on the right, from top to bottom, we have a flying bird, a star, then an abstract anatomical rendition of lungs, heart, and trachea, then a bee, and finally the sacred scarab beetle—our symbol for eternal regeneration. The thing about this is that although I do recognize these symbols, I have never seen them arranged like this and can't decipher what the overall message is. Intuitively, does the cartouche convey anything to either of you?"

"You said that cartouches could express a magical formula," I say. "Well, what if this one is giving us a formula, as in a step-by-step practice? As you said, Karim, the ancients used magic in a practical way to alchemically transform a person into his or her ultimate potential. Well, that sounds a lot like yoga to me. When magic happens, it is always accompanied by a shift in perception. You let go of what you thought was real and find yourself in a more expanded reality. If we are willing to look deeper into this cartouche, perhaps we can see the symbols in a higher light, not as isolated fragments but as pieces of a puzzle. Maybe the symbols indicate a path or a way, a method. Maybe all these years we haven't found yoga in ancient Egypt because the methods weren't written down in the same way they were in India—

maybe they were written more in code and the practitioner had to crack the code. Could it be possible that what is written on this cartouche is a coded formula for a yoga teaching?"

David says, "Really, what Sharon is saying might not be so far-fetched. If you look at many of the classical Indian yogic scriptures, they don't spell everything out in detail; they communicate in the language of riddles. Look at Patanjali's *Yoga Sutras*—short terse statements all strung together. Without commentary by enlightened beings, or at least scholars, it is difficult to make sense out of what Patanjali is saying."

"This is why I wanted to show *you* the cartouche, as I thought you might have an interesting perspective," Karim says. "Tell me, if the cartouche carved on the top of this box could be yoga instructions, do you have any ideas about what that teaching might be and whether it would be relevant to anyone in our time?"

"Karim, do you have a copy of the cartouche I could have? Right now, I only have a hunch and will need more time to contemplate the hieroglyphs, so a photo will be helpful."

"Yes, of course," Karim replies.

Later that evening, back at the hotel, I study the cartouche, going over and over all that had been said during our meeting with Karim. Racking my brain, I rethink the descriptions he gave for each of the images in the cartouche but without coming up with any insights as to a possible connection to yoga, the exception being the two top symbols—the number 10 and the circle with the dot, which hold my attention. Karim said there is a double meaning in the symbol 10—that it also means a yoke, so could read as "yoga." Then Akhenaten's mysterious circle with a dot in the center, hmm . . . This, I thought, could be a pictorial depiction of the atman, the eternal soul within, along with a neat, esoteric teaching describing the aim of yoga: to realize the divine within. The fact that the pharaoh was adamant about God being "One" and that he felt his body was a container for that "One Truth" has got to be significant.

In my mind I hear my teachers' words: God dwells within you, yoga is the journey within; yoga is the realization of the oneness of being; the true Self exists beyond the body and mind. I continue to muse on these concepts, when David reminds me, "Sharon, we have a big day tomorrow, remember we planned a trip to the Pharaonic Village, so don't stay up too late if you want to get up early enough to meditate and do your other yoga practices. The taxi comes at ten."

"Okay, thanks, but I'll be fine."

As David says good night, my mind goes back to the cartouche and I ask myself if there is a yoga teaching there after all. It is possible that I could stretch the ten and the dotted circle to coincide with yoga, but what about those other images? Unable to come up with an answer, I go to bed.

I wake up before the alarm goes off, feeling refreshed and in a great mood, and so grateful to be in Egypt, "Thank you, God!" I say out loud. As I remain lying in the soft, luxurious bed I start remembering all the wonderful people in my life who have been so kind and generous, and one by one I send them a blessing as I see their images float before my mind's eye.

After some minutes I get out of bed and open a window. There's a little ledge where over the past few days I've been leaving bread crumbs and some seeds for the birds. I roll out my yoga mat and start my practice of the Magic Ten, the series of ten asanas that I can usually do in about ten minutes, and follow that with some simple dance steps and breathing exercises. Afterward, I sit down and close my eyes for meditation and place the picture of the cartouche on the floor nearby, hoping perhaps to receive some psychic message. After completing my rounds of japa on my beads, I open my eyes to look at the picture of the cartouche. It is then that I see it—as plain as one would see a bird fly past a window. I see my own morning sadhana, notated, encoded in the ten hieroglyphs of the cartouche—a pharaonic message that had been buried for ages, finally coming to light.

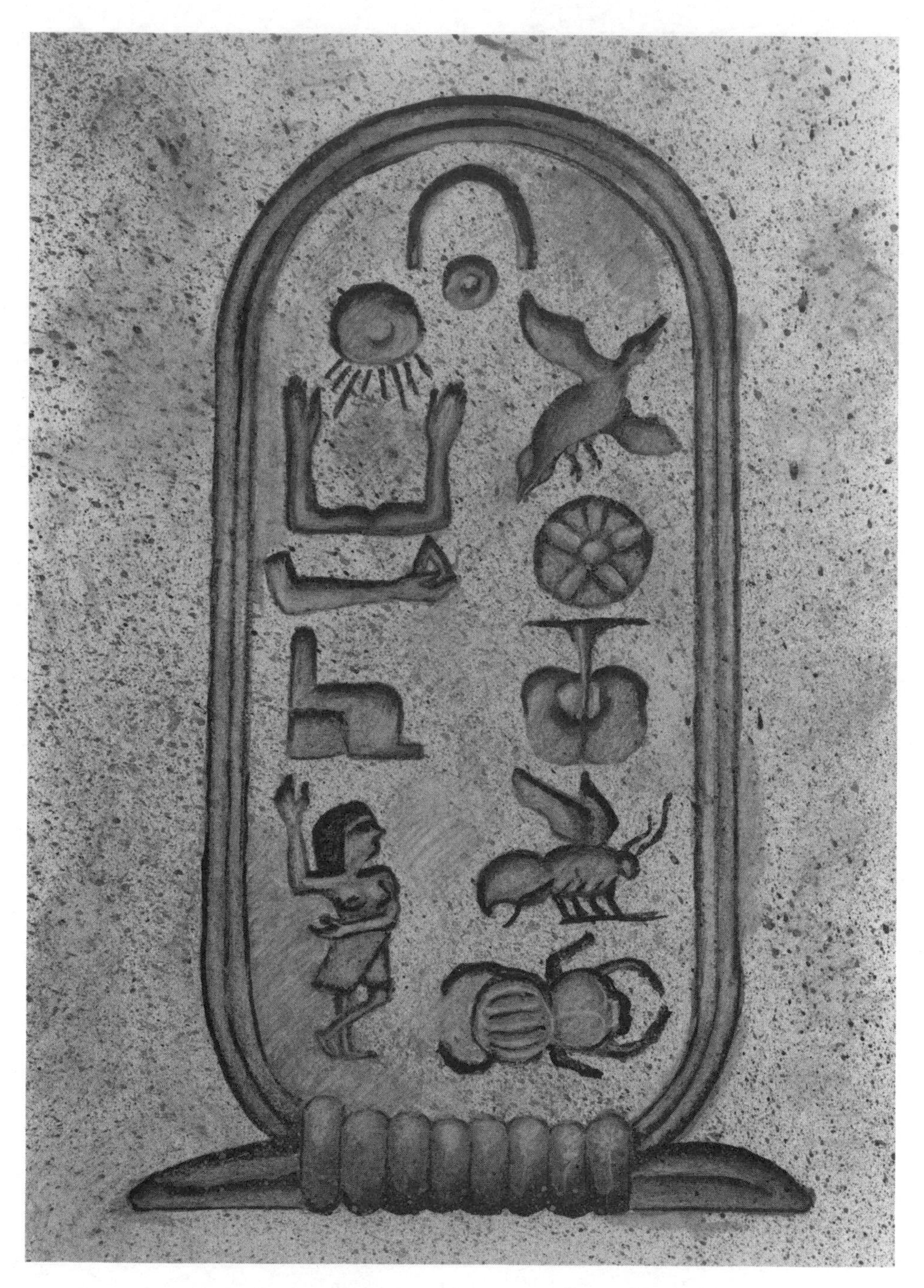

The cartouche showing the coded version of the yogi's way—
The Magic Ten and Beyond

AFTERWORD

IF YOU WANT TO CONVEY something profound, it is often necessary to weave the threads of truth into an engaging story. An important aspect of keeping a spiritual practice attractive and vital is the cultivation of imagination, because through imagination the world becomes a more magical place. A world without magic is mundane and dull. Yoga is magic because the practices shift your perception of yourself and the world beyond the ordinary.

You may or not believe that I found my Magic Ten and Beyond carved in hieroglyphs on an ancient Egyptian cartouche. Does it really matter? When I ask myself, "Where did the Magic Ten and Beyond come from?" I am hard put to cite one authoritative source. When I ask myself where the ideas and images in my mind come from, I have to say they're from my own experiences, remembered—both actual and virtual—and that includes a vast collective that encompasses many minds, not just my own.

Perhaps the brilliant researcher in parapsychology, Dr. Rupert Sheldrake, known for his concept of morphic resonance, can lend some insight here. His hypothesis is that memory is inherent in nature and that there exists a collective memory that all species of life on Earth can tap into. My teacher Shri Brahmananda Saraswati taught that our bodies and minds actually act much like televisions or radios, in that they are able to receive and transmit information. This suggests that our physical selves are actually conduits for vast information systems. Yoga practices help us to focus our minds and develop our ability to magically tap into frequencies beyond those of normal sense perception. Intelligence can be measured by how well one is able to make connections, to link things together. *Yoga* means "to link," and yoga is an intelligent design.

When I ask myself, "Where did yoga come from?" I imagine that yoga could have come from many sources. It seems too big to be just the product of one human civilization. From the beginning, a yogi was known as a free agent, someone who stood outside man's dictates, a truth seeker who strove to live in peaceful harmony with the world. The evidence suggests that, throughout history, yoga practices were always in conflict with the memes of civilization, which do not promote peaceful coexistence. We can observe in our present time how yoga offers a radical departure from the mainstream ideology of our modern lifestyle, which rigidly controls the body through fashion and strict customs that dictate how one should behave with others—other humans, animals, and the environment. Culture has always sought to control our minds and win us over by inciting fear, envy, and greed. We have only to glance at the advertisements that fill our Internet sidebars to see how we are being fed a steady diet of images that appeal to our basest natures.

The mission statement of our worldwide culture could be summed up with the phrase "The Earth belongs to us." Our way of life is founded upon an assumption that being human gives us the right to dominate others—all others, and even Earth herself. Most of us do not question this supposition and feel it is our God-given right to pursue immediate personal happiness, regardless of the consequences to others or the cost to the environment. Yoga has always challenged this assumption.

I imagine that yoga practices were developed around the same time as the seeds of our present culture were being planted, roughly ten thousand years ago. The early civilizations that developed in both ancient Egypt and India were farming cultures in which the enslavement of animals, especially cows, played a central role. The birth of culture coincided with the enslavement of animals. From the enslavement of animals, farming evolved, then slaughterhouses, marketplaces, cities, money, and formal religions. Throughout history and up to the present day, culture has advocated a way of life that takes essentially a "might is right" approach, expressed as the right of the strongest or richest to take what they want from whomever they want. Our laws tell us that if we own it, we have the right to use it in whatever way we want. This unchallenged attitude of privilege allows us to use others without concern for their well-being, happiness, or freedom. We have been waging war on other human beings for longer than we can count the years, and underlying that is the war we have been waging against Mother Nature and the animals for even longer. All wars, past and present, violence, enslavement, and exploitation have been waged beneath the banner of peace and happiness. Violence never brings peace or happiness—it only brings more violence. Yoga has always offered a way to true peace and happiness. The true history (or *her-story*) of yoga has yet to be revealed to us, and when it is it will most likely be beyond our wildest imagining. Will it be imagining? Or will it be remembering?

I like to think that while the way of our present culture was being established ten thousand years ago, there were a few rare human beings who stood apart and looked upon what was happening with a critical, reflective eye. They did not see war, slavery, exploitation, and the accumulation of material wealth as the way to lasting happiness. So they rejected the ways of civilization and retreated into the wild places—the mountains, deserts, jungles, and forests—to discover the way to real happiness on their own. Removed from civilization they could experiment with ways to increase happiness that did not depend on hurting others or depriving them of happiness. The stories found in ancient scriptures refer to those beings as *rishis*, sages, or yogis—men and women who lived in harmony with nature and seemed to possess an illuminated, otherworldly self-confidence that was not dependent on material wealth, dominance over or control of others, or religious rituals but rested in their direct connection to the transcendental source of happiness itself—God, the Supreme Divine and Eternal One.

Those early yogis felt that human arrogance actually came from an ego gone out of control. The ego is incapable of compassion—a person ruled by ego stoops to any cruelty in the hopes of getting ahead. These early yogis honed practices that increased humility and compassion, enabling them to shift their sense of identity away from the ego and its selfish demands for satisfaction. Once freed of selfishness they could delve deeper into the search for truth and reconnect to the eternal, blissful Self within. Over time, these magical practices came to be known as yoga.

Perhaps some of those ancient yogis have reincarnated and are walking among us today, when we are in the midst of a universal environmental and spiritual crisis. I think yoga is so popular in the world today because Earth needs yogis—those who know how to live in harmony with her. These practices provide us with ways to transform ourselves and the world into a magical place. The yogi's way is the way of kindness and compassion and is available to us now—to anyone who has the courage to dare to care about the happiness of others.

GLOSSARY

(Most words are Sanskrit unless otherwise indicated)

ABHINIVESHA: fear of death; one of the five kleshas or obstacles to Yoga, cited by Patanjali in the *Yoga Sutras*

ABHYASA: sadhana, practice, to sit with something over a long period of time; continuous effort, repeated endeavor

AGNI: fire

AJNA: to perceive; sixth chakra, third eye center

AKHENATEN: (1353–1336 BCE) a pharaoh of Egypt of the Eighteenth Dynasty, ruler of Egypt for seventeen years; previously known as Amenhotep IV. He founded the city of Amarna, moving the capital from Thebes. Known as the heretic king because he instituted the first known monotheistic religion in the world.

ASANA: seat, connection to the Earth, relationship to the Earth and all beings.

ASHTANGA: eight-limbed. The eight-step path of raja yoga as described by Patanjali: yama, niyama, asana, pranayama, pratyahara, dharana, dhyana, samadhi; the name of the system of yoga taught by Shri K. Pattabhi Jois

ANAHATA: unstruck; fourth chakra, heart center

ANTU: may it be so

ATMAN: the eternal soul, the True Self, which dwells within every being

AVIDYA: ignorance; mis-knowing; mistaking the unreal for the real; one of the five kleshas or obstacles to Yoga, cited by Patanjali

BANDHA: from the verb root *bandh*, meaning to bind; a bandha is an energetic lock, used to direct the flow of prana

BHAKTI: from the root *bhaj*, meaning to treat with reverence, affection, and love; devotion to God

BHAV(A): blissful divine mood of unitive consciousness; to directly experience love for God; enlightened emotional perception, feeling, or mood connected to the divine

BRAHMA: the one who expands; the creator of the universe

CARTOUCHE: a French word meaning "gun cartridge." When Napoleon's soldiers came to Egypt in the late 1700s, they saw many of these shapes enclosing hieroglyphic writings. At the time no one could read hieroglyphs and they did not know what they were looking at; but to them they looked like empty bullet cartridges. The word became so commonly used that it has remained the standard term for describing the oval ring encircled with a pictorial representation of a rope folded and tied at the end, usually containing a name written in Egyptian hieroglyphs. Before the shape was elongated it was a circle and was called a *sheni*, meaning "to encircle," but in order to fit more hieroglyphs inside, the circle was stretched into an oval shape.

CHAKRA: wheel, circle; doorway of perception

CHITTA: mind stuff, thoughts, fluctuations, whirlings

CHITTA PRASADANAM: a mind with a sweet disposition

DEVO MAHESWARA: a name for Lord Shiva, the destructive aspect of the Hindu Trinity

DHARANA: concentration, the ability to focus the mind leading to dhyana or meditation

DHYANA: the meditative state of absorption; the continuous focus of attention on one object without interruption

DIVINE: transcendental, beyond the mundane, temporal world; heavenly; celestial

GURU: the remover of darkness/ignorance; spiritual teacher

HARE: invocative of Hara, a name for Radha, Krishna's consort (or Shakti)

HARI: a name for Krishna, which means the one who removes all afflictions

HATHA YOGA: from the root *hath*, meaning "to force." Hatha yoga is the yoga of force. Ha = sun + tha = moon; a practice for balancing the pairs of opposites—sun/moon, right/left, male/female, self/other

HATHA YOGA PRADIPIKA: The title of an ancient technical manual written in sutra form, by yogi Swatmarama in the fourteenth century. The title means "Shedding light on how to join together the sun and the moon."

IDA: the white moon stream; left nadi; receptive channel

JAPA: repetition of mantra

JIVA: individual soul, the embodied self separate from others

JIVANMUKTA: a liberated soul

JIVAMUKTI: living liberated

KAPALABHATI: skull shining

KARMA: action. According to the law of karma, one's current situation is the result of his or her past actions.

KECHARI MUDRA: a yogic seal, used in kriya and pranayama practices, in which the tip of the tongue is curled back and pressed upward against the soft palate, a position designed to awaken spiritual energies by quieting the tongue, and diminishing hunger, unnecessary speech, and distracting thoughts

KLESHA: obstacle. Patanjali in the *Yoga Sutras* lists five kleshas, or obstacles to yoga: *avidya* (ignorance), *asmita* (egoism), *raga* (likes), *dvesa* (aversions), and *abhinivesha* (fear of death)

KRISHNA: The most attractive, one's innermost heart's desire; black; dark; the Supreme Self; God

KRIYA: purification action

KUMBHAK(A): to hold; savor

KUNDALINI: consciousness, said to lie in a dormant state, coiled like a snake at the base of the spine in the muladhara chakra. As enlightenment begins to dawn, consciousness as kundalini starts to ascend upward through the chakras in the central channel.

LEELA: cosmic play, the Eternal Divine drama

LOKAH: location, place, world, realm

MALA: rosary; prayer beads strung together and used for reciting mantras and prayers

MAMA: mine

MANIPURA: the jewel in the city, third chakra

MANTRA: protection for the mind. From man = mind + tra = to cross over

MARG(A): path, way

MUDRA: energy seal, used to direct prana in a particular way. Mudras are usually performed as hand gestures, but there are also mudras that are done with the whole body.

MULA: root

MULADHARA: root place; first chakra, at the base of the spine

NADI: channel, river, current, stream; energetic conduit for prana, life force

NAMAH: not me—I bow to a higher Self

OM: the pranava, that which ever renews itself; the primal name of God. The three most basic sounds that a human being can make: AH-OO-MM.

PADMASANA: lotus seat, performed by lifting your right foot and placing it high on your left inner thigh, then lifting your left foot and placing it high on your right thigh; traditionally one of the suggested seats for pranayama and meditation practice.

PARAM: beyond, highest, best

PATANJALI: The name of the author of the *Yoga Sutras*, who lived roughly two thousand to five thousand years ago. The name means: pa (falling snake) + anjali (open hands). The legend says that he fell as a snake into the waiting hands of his mother and so he was called Patanjali.

PHARAOH: (Greek) originally from the root *pr* meaning "house + great," referring to a palace; but from the time of Akhenaten, the word was used as a title for the king or ruler of Egypt.

PINGALA: the red sun stream, the right nadi, masculine channel

PRANA: life force, vitality; one of the five vayus or winds. Prana vayu is the upward-moving wind.

PRANAYAMA: from prana = life force + yama = restrict; to restrict the life force, or, pran + ayama = to expand or set free the life force

PRASAD: a gracious, blessed gift, something that has been offered to God or to a respected person, then given back to the giver; a term used often with regard to food that has been offered.

PUSHTI: well nourished, graceful

PUSHTI MARG: path of grace, a yogic lineage founded by Shri Vallabhacharya (1479–1531)

RAMA: pronounced with a long "a," Rama means the avatar of Vishnu, the hero of the Ramayana epic. Pronounced with a short "a," Rama is another name for Laxmi, the goddess of fortune.

SADHANA: conscious spiritual practice; action done with the intention to realize Yoga

SAHASRARA: thousand-petaled; seventh or crown chakra, located above the top of the head

SAKSHAT: nearby

SAKSHI: witness

SAMA: same, steady, neutral, equal, calm

SAMADHI: same as the highest; enlightenment; Yoga; connection with God; the eighth limb of Patanjali's Ashtanga yoga system

SAMASTA: same standing

SARA: to wash or agitate

SARCOPHAGI: (Greek) stone coffers

SATCHIDANANDA: truth, consciousness, and bliss; the attributes of the eternal and supreme Divine Self

SATTVA: light, pure, balanced

SHAKTI: female principle of divine energy

SHANTI: peace, calmness

SHARANAM: refuge, sanctuary, safe place

SHAVASANA: the seat of the corpse; the practice of dying, of letting go of the physical body

SHIVA: auspicious one

SHRI: divinely beautiful

STHIRA: steady, stable, consistent

SUKHA: "sweet space"; comfortable, spacious, ease, a sense of lightness and joy

SUKHINOH: happy, at ease, comfortable

SWADHISTHANA: Her favorite standing place; second chakra

TAMASIC: sluggish, dark, decaying

UDDIYANA BANDHA: flying-up lock, done by lifting the diaphragm upward after exhaling

VAYU: air, wind, vital force

VIRASANA: hero seat; a yogic asana where the practitioner sits down between both feet with knees together; a suggested seat used for pranayama and meditation practice

VISHNU: the Supreme Lord; the all-pervading reality and sustainer of the universe

VISHUDDHA: place of purity; poison free; fifth chakra

YOGA: (capitalized) yoke, join, connect, remember; union with the Self, with God; enlightenment

YOGA: (lower case) the practices, which are intended to bring about Yoga, or enlightenment.

YOGI: one who has remembered God; one who is united with the higher Self, with God; one who has attained Yoga, or enlightenment; one who practices yoga

ACKNOWLEDGMENTS

Thank you, **David Life**, for your ongoing creative partnership and support, which manifests in a multitude of ways, including the wonderful drawings you provided for the book, as well as the book's design concept. The many hours you spent listening to me read aloud from the early manuscript, giving me feedback and encouraging me to write the Egyptian adventure story. And always without complaint, patiently coming to my assistance when I needed help solving computer issues while writing.

They say a picture is worth a thousand words, so if this book had no pictures it would have to have many more pages filled with many more words and most likely be quite dull. So I must thank **Constance Hansen** and **Russell Peacock**, the dynamic duo known as **Guzman**, for saving us from dullness with their illustrative photographs.

Thank you to my editor, **Sara Carder**, at TarcherPerigee, for believing that my personal yogic way could also be of benefit to others and for seeing my book as akin to Julia Cameron's *The Artist's Way*. Also thank you to **Heather Brennan** and the publishing team for caring and for supporting me along every step of the way. I am deeply indebted to **Megan Newman** for introducing me to Sara.

I would feel very alone without the support of my trusted literary agent, **Joel Gotler**, who expertly navigates our ship through the rough waters and stormy seas of the publishing world as well as knowing when to float, all the while with compass in hand, never losing sight of the direction we are headed.

Much appreciation to Jivamukti Yoga teacher and registered nurse, the brilliant

Cassandra Rigney, for her expertise and insights in regard to the physiological effects of kapalabhati and pranayama upon the lungs and kidneys.

I joyfully acknowledge my dear friend, the respected physicist and Egyptologist **Tommy Broussard**, for seriously listening to my theory. Many years ago, when I asked Tommy if he thought yoga could have been practiced in ancient Egypt, he said he didn't know but if anyone did it would be his friend, the charismatic **Zahi Hawass,** who, it turned out, was at the time none other than the Egyptian Minister of State for Antiquities. At that time Dr. Hawass rejected the idea and told Tommy to tell me that there was no way yoga could have been practiced in ancient Egypt. But recently, while I was at work on this manuscript, Tommy reported to me that he had talked with Dr. Hawass, who said, "At first I dismissed your friend the yoga teacher's theory, but some evidence has surfaced that may support her idea; but it would still be very hard to prove." Anyway, I must credit both Tommy and Dr. Hawass for giving me the inspiration for the fictitious character of Karim Hassan.

I bow to my guru-ji, **Shri K. Pattabhi Jois**, for his sense of adventure and often mischievous and mysterious ways. When Pattabhi Jois was asked how his system of Ashtanga Yoga came about—specifically where the asana series came from—he said that one day when he was with his guru, Shri Krishnamacharya, in the Calcutta Library they came upon a long-lost yoga text written on banana leaves, pictorially showing all of the asana sequences. When I asked if I could see those leaves, he laughed and replied, "The ants have eaten them a long time ago!"

I am always grateful to my ballet teacher, the great **Ruthanna Boris**. When I lived in Seattle, Washington, studying with Ms. Boris from 1973 to 1979, she taught the class a series of warm-up exercises that she referred to as the "magic seven." She assured us that all the dancers at the New York City Ballet practiced the magic seven every morning before they did their first pliés at the barre. She told us that Joseph Pilates himself had taught it to the company as a warm-up for the dancers, one that would help safeguard them against injuries. I don't remember the whole series, but I do remember that it included a modified shoulder-stand and that this was probably my first encounter with a yoga asana. The idea to put the word "magic" into my own series of warm-up exercises certainly can be traced back to Ms. Boris's magic seven.

Gratitude to **Kathleen Hunt**, who practiced the magic seven alongside me for many years with Ruthanna Boris while we were dance students together at the University of Washington in the 1970s. It was with Kathleen that I shared an interest in Napoleonic French history, and it was she who encouraged me to include a handstand in my morning yoga practice and inspired me, through her own disciplined example, to gradually increase the time I spent standing on my hands every morning, so that now I am up to a sixty-breath handstand.

Thank you to **Kelly Britton**, **Rob Fraboni**, **Giacobazzi Yanez**, **Carly Boland**, **Arjun Bruggeman**, **Alex Febre**, **Hari Mulukutla**, **Katya Grineva**, **DeAnna Haun**, and **Steven Haun** for patiently listening to me read the early version of the manuscript and for providing suggestions to make the text read more smoothly. Much appreciation goes to **Jaimie Epstein** and **Katie Manitsas** for their helpful editing assistance early on in the developing manuscript.

I continue to be deeply moved by all the **Jivamukti Yoga students** who, over the years, have found the Magic Ten series of ten simple exercises to be of benefit to them. I hope that with this new book, they will embrace the expanded version of the Magic Ten, adding the "beyond" additions to their own daily personal practice.

ABOUT THE AUTHOR

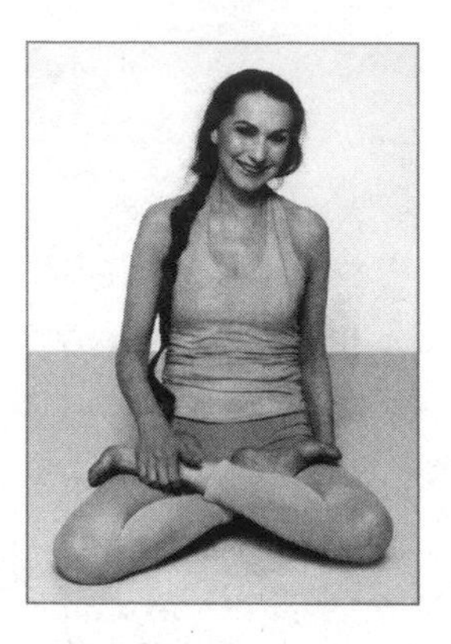

SHARON GANNON, author, musician, animal rights/vegan activist, is the co-creator, along with David Life, of the Jivamukti Yoga method, a path to enlightenment through compassion for all beings.

www.jivamuktiyoga.com
www.simplerecipesforjoy.com